Complete Guide and Toolkit
to Successful
EHR Adoption

Jeffery Daigrepont, EFMP, CAPPM

Debra McGrath, CRNP

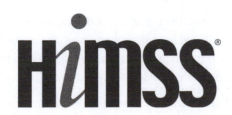

HIMSS Mission

To lead healthcare transformation through the effective use of health information technology.

Printed in the U.S.A. 5 4 3 2 1

Requests for permission to make copies of any part of this work should be sent to:
Permissions Editor
HIMSS
230 E. Ohio, Suite 500
Chicago, IL 60611-3270
nvitucci@himss.org

ISBN: 978-0-9821070-9-6

For more information about HIMSS, please visit www.himss.org.

About the Authors

Jeffery Daigrepont, EFMP, CAPPM, has over 20 years of consulting experience in healthcare technology, operations, revenue cycle management, compliance, stimulus funding and strategic planning for hospitals and physician practices. As one of the nation's leading experts in electronic health records (EHRs), Mr. Daigrepont has helped over 5,000 physicians successfully adopt EHR systems from various vendors. The American Medical Association (AMA), HIMSS and numerous media outlets have called on his guidance and input. Regarded as a go-to source for top-tier media, he serves on national committees and as a keynote speaker at various national healthcare conferences. Mr. Daigrepont is the author of the AMA's *Starting a Medical Practice, Second Edition* and *Automating the Medical Record*, and Greenbranch Publishing's *The Complete EMR Selection Guide*.

Daigrepont developed and managed the national health IT service line—procuring and implementing over $500M in health IT-related services throughout the United States for the Coker Group, a nationally recognized healthcare consulting firm that provides hospitals, physician practices and other providers with innovative, principled solutions in business operations, finance and IT to help them achieve their optimum level of productivity. Through ESSENCE Healthcare, Mr. Daigrepont is responsible for strategy and business development of their technology companies offered to members, which includes ClearPractice, a wholly owned subsidiary.

Daigrepont is an active member of the Healthcare Information and Management Systems Society (HIMSS) and is credentialed by the American Academy of Medical Management (AAMM) with an Executive Fellowship in Practice Management (EFMP) and Certified Administrator in Physician Practice Management (CAPPM).

Debra McGrath, CRNP, Senior Vice President, heads the Coker Group's Technology service line. With a primary focus on clinical information technology, her role includes oversight of technology acquisition, implementation and utilization in the ambulatory and inpatient setting. Under her oversight, the company provides technology support services to practices and healthcare entities across the nation.

A Perinatal Clinical Nurse Specialist and experienced Nurse Practitioner, Ms. McGrath spent much of her career in nursing before moving into management, and has dedicated years to healthcare-related academic pursuits. She is an expert on applications in ambulatory settings, federally qualified and community health centers, nurse practitioner practice, patient data collection, warehousing and reporting, and handheld and wireless technologies.

Ms. McGrath holds a BSN from West Chester University, an MSN in Perinatal Nursing, University of Pennsylvania, and a Post-Master's Certificate as a Family Nurse Practitioner, Wilmington College. She is Board Certified in Family Practice, American

Nursing Credentialing Center. She is a well-published author and experienced speaker presenting for associations and organizations throughout the country.

ABOUT THE CONTRIBUTING AUTHOR

Gabriel Harry is a seasoned information technology professional bringing 10 years of technology experience to the healthcare industry. Mr. Harry began his career in 1996 as a medical biller with Equifax Risk Management, billing hospital claims for several healthcare systems in the Southeast region. As a client service manager, his responsibilities for managing integrated billing systems grew his enthusiasm for technology and led him to pursue his Bachelor's of Science Degree in Network and Data Communications. While at Pennsylvania College of Technology, he supported the faculty, staff and laboratory environments of the Health Science and Technology Schools. Upon graduation, Mr. Harry returned to Atlanta, Georgia, where he continued consulting with private practice physicians and groups in project management, implementation, upgrading and deployment of Practice Management and Electronic Medical Records Systems. His projects have encompassed Wide Area Networks integration, data center upgrades/hosting, support desk staffing, database migrations, and staff training. With a passion for technology, Mr. Harry is a candidate for a Master's Degree in Healthcare Information Systems.

Dedication

This book is dedicated to all the early adopters, visionaries and pioneers of electronic health records.

Acknowledgments

We would like to give special thanks to the Healthcare Information and Management Systems Society (HIMSS) for the opportunity to write this book. We especially thank Fran Perveiler, Vice President, Communications, for her guidance and input on the book design and content. Also, we thank Mary Griskewicz, Senior Director, Ambulatory Information Systems, for giving us access to her vast network of subject matter experts. Nancy Vitucci, Manager, Publications, has been patient and tireless in putting this book together in a professional way. Thank you all.

Contents

Preface

As of the writing of this book, more than 10 years have passed since the infamous report by the Institute of Medicine (IOM) called for a national effort to make healthcare safer through the use of electronic health records (EHRs). Since this time, EHRs have been poised to be the answer to many of the challenges facing our nation's healthcare delivery system. Stakeholders from every corner have been involved in the complex challenge of working toward automation. The field encompasses innovative physicians, distinguished policy leaders, members of congress, major corporations, trade associations, nurses, office managers, executives and three presidential administrations—including Presidents Clinton, Bush, and Obama.

A renewed surge occurred during the George W. Bush administration with the appointment of Dr. David Brailer as the National Health Information Technology Coordinator on April 27, 2004. Dr. Brailer's office was responsible for the creation of an interoperable, standards-based Nationwide Health Information Network in support of President Bush's goal to establish the widespread adoption of electronic healthcare records within 10 years. The American National Standards Institute received one of the contract awards to fund the Healthcare Information Technology Standards Panel. The Panel's mission was to assist in the development of a Nationwide Health Information Network by addressing the standards-related issues impacting the harmonization of healthcare data and networks. During this era, some of the first laws were passed allowing hospitals to financially subsidize the cost of an EHR to their medical staff. Dr. Brailer served for two years.

The election of President Barack Obama brought sweeping new incentives to the decade-long challenge of getting physicians to adopt EHRs. Of the nearly $800 billion American Recovery and Reinvestment Act (ARRA), $22 billion was earmarked for the advancement of healthcare information technology, including EHRs. As a part of the ARRA stimulus bill, eligible providers (EP) that see a certain percentage of Medicare or Medicaid patients are eligible to receive incentives of $44,000 to $66,000 for adopting EHRs. Those that do not adopt EHRs will see reductions in their Medicare reimbursement.

Despite all the efforts, adoption of EHRs in the Unites States remains extremely low according to most studies. Even with the introduction of stimulus incentives, many physicians are unsure or unwilling to adopt. Furthermore, those with EHRs report not using them or they complain that the software does not work at the point of care. For many, the reward of an EHR may seem ambiguous when contrasting the cost of adopting and the amount of training required to learn the system. When benefits are not seen immediately, it can be easy to give up, especially if using the EHR makes running the practice more costly. However, when implemented correctly, *with the right vendor,*

EHRs can make a profoundly positive impact on any practice, including improving profitability and patient care.

Regardless of where you are in your journey of either adopting a new EHR or trying to optimize an existing EHR, the *Complete Guide and Toolkit to Successful EHR Adoption* will walk you through the process in a practical, easy-to-follow way with proven strategies to ensure success. You will learn proven methods for ensuring the selection of the right vendor and for holding the vendor accountable for meeting its obligations. This book covers critical success factors for implementing and optimizing an EHR as well as provides easy-to-use assessment tools to assist with making important decisions. Additionally, it addresses complicated federal standards and policies to ensure that each reader fully understands compliance requirements and the opportunities to take advantage of financial incentives.

HOW TO USE THIS BOOK

Rather than reading this book one time and putting it away, the user will want to regard this book as a flight plan and refer to it frequently. As a flight plan for the EHR journey, the following areas are addressed.

- **Phase I – Groundwork.** This is the starting point, when you gather essential requirements necessary for your journey. Are all your systems working? Do you have enough fuel? Are all your team members on board and ready to go?
- **Phase II – Boarding.** You now have to get everything settled into its right place, secure and ready for takeoff, just as passengers do by taking their seats, storing luggage, and buckling up. In the case of an EHR journey, this could mean taking corrective action to any threats discovered during the groundwork, similar to a captain who calls in maintenance to correct a problem before takeoff.
- **Phase III – Takeoff.** Now things are getting exciting and even a little scary. Everything is moving fast; some of your passengers are starting to get nervous. This is when all your preparation work starts to pay off. Your subject matter experts are prepared to answer questions, and, if necessary, you have appropriate preparations for anyone who is sick over the transformation.
- **Phase IV – During the Flight.** This is when things start to get interesting and you may even encounter unexpected turbulence, disorderly passengers and an in-flight diversion to get around a storm cloud. At this stage, you are thinking about grabbing the parachute but, with a little confidence, you will get through it. This book addresses dealing with the human behavior side of change management and provides strategies for dealing with these challenges.
- **Phase V – Landing.** As most experts will say, this is the most critical phase of the journey; in EHR vernacular, we call this "go live." How you ultimately land or go live will determine if you are able to move on to future destinations. This book provides proven strategies for making sure you have a smooth landing.
- **Phase VI – Future Destination.** Now that you have landed with success, it is time to look at what is next. This is a good time to start thinking about optimization and tweaking your existing system for improvements. This book guides you through optimization taking your EHR to the next level.

So get a pen, highlighter and notepad. Do not be afraid to mark up this book, highlighting important points and making notes. Use it as a guide for the journey as you lead your practice through this transformation. Have fun along the way, and do not be afraid to challenge the "stonewallers." Be prepared to make changes and adjust your strategies as needed. While this book offers great suggestions, every situation creates unique challenges and opportunities. Some of the best decisions will come from trial and error and from unexpected sources.

An EHR transformation will touch virtually every aspect of your practice and bring about an entirely new way of thinking and doing business. The benefits far outweigh the cost of doing nothing, which includes the risk of becoming technologically isolated from consumers, payers and others in the healthcare community. While no system is perfect, and no time will ever be the perfect time to adopt an EHR, most agree that healthcare must be automated to meet future challenges. We hope this book provides you with the information necessary to be successful with EHR adoption and optimization.

Jeffery Daigrepont, EFMP, CAPPM, and Debra McGrath, CRNP

Are You Ready for the Electronic Health Records Journey?

THE EARLY YEARS

Health information technology (IT) has changed exponentially over the past decade. Understanding where the industry has been will help readers understand and appreciate the many strategies throughout this book and provide some insight to where we have been and where we are going in the ever-changing health IT landscape.

In the late 1970s to early 1980s, the healthcare industry was slowly becoming electronic. Up until that point, paper peg-board systems were used for billing, paper appointment books captured scheduling and paper charts were used for collecting and storing clinical information.

Most of the vendors during this era only sold UNIX-based practice management systems and hospital information systems with limited ability to store clinical data. UNIX is a type of operating system that pre-dates Microsoft Windows®. These systems were sometimes referred to as charter-based systems or "green screens" because they were not as graphical as what we see today. Nearly all insurance claims were recorded on paper and sent by mail because we did not have electronic clearinghouses to transmit claims. Reports were printed on dot matrix printers using the old "green bar" or "track" paper. In some cases, reports could take up to 24 hours to run. Those who recall any of this can appreciate the improvements of today's systems.

In the early 1990s, niche vendors with specialty products began to appear on the scene; this eventually developed into vendors with a focus on electronic health records (EHRs), clinical data repositories, clinical decision support and data warehousing products. The term "enterprise" or "fully integrated" had not yet been established, so all vendors had to "play" to co-exist through what is commonly known as interfacing of software or using best-of-breed technology. By co-existing, one vendor provided the practice management (PM) system; another vendor provided the lab system; a third vendor provided the pharmacy system and so on, and so on.

At the Annual Conferences & Exhibitions presented by the Healthcare Information and Management Systems Society (HIMSS) during this era, most of the exhibitors were vendors that only sold software to hospitals, and most of those who attended were chief information officers. Cerner, EPIC, McKesson, Meditech and Siemens were some of the primary vendors selling to hospitals at that time. Very few ambulatory vendors, if any, were exhibiting, and physicians, nurses, chief medical officers (CMOs) and chief executive officers (CEOs) were not in attendance like they are today. On the outpatient/ambulatory vendor side, there were just a handful of solutions. In fact, the majority of the market share was held by three primary vendors: IDX, Medical Manager and Misys. Now, there are more than 600 vendors selling some type of health IT solution to hospitals and physicians.

THE INTERFACING ERA

As stated previously, the majority of the PM systems and hospital information systems (HIS) installed across the United States were developed on UNIX-based technology or in Cobalt, which dates back to the early 1970s. As a result, medical practices buying EHR systems at this time had to interface their EHR system with their PM system or run two separate systems. Interfacing was expensive and complicated because generally two vendors were required to work together, which is not always easy (this era may have spawned the term "finger pointing"). Concerns such as version control, disjointed workflow among the applications and data integrity issues were common. It also required multiple servers, multiple database tables and an interface engine requiring continuous troubleshooting.

Considering all the discrete data elements necessary for delivering safe patient care, it is no wonder why this disjointed approach was unsustainable and, in some cases, unsafe. Important information such as medication was not reconciled between two systems storing information on the same patient. Patient care requires collaboration from multiple caregivers and delivery systems; thus, information must be stored and managed by multiple systems. To illustrate this point, Table 1 shows a list of just a few primary systems and their roles in health IT.

Moving along, in the late 1990s, vendors that had only PM systems or HIS systems started acquiring stand-alone EHR vendors or developing their own EHR technology. The national trend toward vendor consolidation, driven by the market demand for a single vendor solution, was in full swing going into 2000. To avert finger pointing and the complications of expensive interfacing, vendors were evolving into one-stop-shop software providers. A rapid explosion of new vendors entered the market during this period, offering systems built on more modern program languages and robust databases. The Internet was also being leveraged, allowing web-based solutions to enter the market in sufficient numbers and as an alternative to purchasing hardware and software. The application service providers (ASPs) concept was rapidly emerging. By this time, terminology like *fully integrated systems, single vendor solutions* or *one throat the choke* were becoming popular. The term "enterprise vendor" was regarded as the ideal solution for those who wanted to address a wide breadth of needs through a single vendor relationship.

Technology	How It Is Used
Practice Management (PM) Systems	Used by physician offices to schedule appointments, capture charges, post payments and file insurance
Electronic Health Records (EHRs)	Used in both the hospital and physician office to capture clinical information
Computerized Practitioner Order Entry (CPOE)	Used by hospitals to capture orders such as labs, medications and procedures during a patient's hospital stay
Hospital Information Systems (HIS)	Used by hospital offices to manage admissions and discharges, capture charges, post payments and file insurance
Picture Archiving and Communication Systems (PACS)	Used to store digital radiology images such as x-rays, CTs and EKGs
Radiology Information System (RIS)	Used by radiology departments to manage patients' schedules, appointments and billing information
Electronic Prescribing (eRX)	Used to electronically order and manage patient medications.
Document Imaging Management System (DIMS)	Used to manage paper documents by converting scanned documents into PDFs for electronic storage and retrieval.

Table 1: Primary Systems in Health IT

THE ENTERPRISE ERA

Enterprise-wide vendors typically offer multi-product/module solutions for healthcare providers including acute care (inpatient), outpatient, and other modules such as lab information systems and radiology information systems. Some offer more comprehensive packages than others do, but the basic concept is the same—a single vendor/single database solution with all applications integrated into a single solution.

Today there are two types of enterprise vendors:

1. Those that acquired technology through mergers and acquisitions and have consolidated the products into one solution, often through interfacing or sharing a single database. These vendors generally have a lot of flexibility because they can

still sell just a PM system or just an EHR. In other words, they can unbundle their solutions, because the systems offered initially operated as stand-alone products.

2. Those that developed a solution entirely on a single source code, common database with shared tables. These vendors are sometimes referred to as organic enterprise vendors. They are appealing because the entire system is built as one, which is generally an improvement to the workflow within the system.

While enterprise vendors have a lot to offer, interfacing and coexisting with other vendors is still very common, especially with other caregivers or outside databases, such as lab systems, pharmacies, hospitals, etc. The issue of sharing and exchanging data is still a challenge as the market goes from "data collectors" to "data users."

THE CERTIFICATION ERA

As EHRs became increasingly popular, the adoption started to move from early adopters (technology savvy physicians) to what is regarded as the "average users." Early adopters were considered techie physicians who were willing to tolerate some of the shortfalls in technology and who enjoyed participating in the development of EHR technology. The average user, on the other hand, found that EHRs were slowing them down and in some cases, posing a threat to their productivity and incomes. The average user was not interested in writing templates, building drug lists, or programming triggers to enhance their EHRs. The average user just wanted to buy a system, plug it in, and use it. However, the technology still required a lot of customizing and formatting around functionality necessary to use an EHR at the point of care.

A significant amount of movement transpired during this era; unfortunately, it was not all forward movement. While adoption was becoming popular, EHR failures and de-installs were also on the rise. Many physicians that purchased EHRs quickly had buyer's remorse and gave up altogether. EHR failures were not uncommon and there were concerns over the cost to adopt. Members of the Medical Group Management Association (MGMA) reported spending as much as $32,600 per physician to adopt an EHR.[1]

The vendor industry was profiting nicely because the physician usually did not have the time or technical skill to do his or her own customizing. Customization service was outsourced to expensive consultants and/or back to the vendor for an extra fee. Lack of standards and inconsistent collaboration programming development among vendors were contributing to this challenge. To be fair, many practices were reluctant to change behavior and many were attempting to make their EHRs work in the same way as a paper chart. To make matters worse, the approach to implementing was an "all or nothing" approach, where the vendor and practice attempted to install everything at once. Today, it is done in stages and phases—allowing everyone to adjust to the changes.

To address these challenges, organizations such as the American Health Information Management Association (AHIMA), HIMSS, and The National Alliance for Health Information Technology (Alliance) provided the initial capital contributions to form a certification commission as an independent 501(c)3 nonprofit organization limited liability corporation, known today as the Certification Commission for Health Information Technology (CCHIT).

The intent of CCHIT is to influence EHR functionality, development, and design as a way to foster improvements in quality, safety, efficiency and access—key goals in today's national dialog on health reform. Founded in 2004, and certifying EHRs since 2006, the Commission established the first comprehensive, practical definition of what capabilities were needed in these systems. The certification criteria were developed through a voluntary, consensus-based process engaging diverse stakeholders, and the federal government officially recognized CCHIT as a certifying body.

THE DATA DRIVEN MARKET

As a result of the above, the industry is now moving into the era of health information exchange (HIE) or sharing. Past attempts at this were known as regional health information organizations (RHIOs). RHIOs were difficult to sustain financially, and in most cases, offered little value to caregivers or patients because only a handful of stakeholders were participating; this left many gaps in the continuity of data. Furthermore, there was rarely a business case or economic justification for participating. While everyone agrees sharing data can improve patient care, without incentives, justifying the cost and effort was difficult. Additionally, some RHIOs were becoming data islands, and in some cases, unintentionally isolating some stakeholders who had systems unable to conform to standards. As a result, the last several years have been consumed with an extensive focus on industry standards and compliance around exchanging and sharing information. Along with the help of HIMSS, vendors have been collaborating and willing to align their solutions to enable data sharing across different systems.

WHERE DO WE GO FROM HERE?

The question "where do we go from here" is frequently heard in speeches, articles, health IT think tanks, and among stakeholders trying to sort out how they position their organizations for the future. This question brings to mind a quote from *Alice's Adventures in Wonderland*.[2]

> "Would you tell me, please, which way I ought to go from here?"
> "That depends a good deal on where you want to get to," said the Cat.
> "I don't much care where," said Alice.
> "Then it doesn't matter which way you go," said the Cat.
> "—so long as I get SOMEWHERE," Alice added as an explanation.
> "Oh, you're sure to do that," said the Cat, "if you only walk long enough."

While no one can completely predict the future with accuracy, a few trends are becoming clear. First, the industry will continue to move away from best-of-breed systems and toward fully integrated single vendor solutions. This initiative will be driven and accelerated out of the need to meet federal compliance requirements and data reporting requirements. Systems that incorporate the functionality of patient registration, scheduling, and billing combined with the functionality of documenting a patient's clinical visit and ensuring follow-up for health-promotion and disease-prevention activities will be essential. Many of the top-tier vendors have already adopted this strategy through acquisitions or internal development of EHRs. Second, industry standards and the need to conform and comply with federal mandates will continue to become more complex, which will likely force smaller vendors out of business and/or into merging with more established vendors. The third movement is toward consumer participation and provider portals that provide direct, secure access to patient-level information to the patient and referring providers. Further, patient portals help practices become more efficient by allowing patients direct access for scheduling and entering their medical, surgical, and social histories. Secure portals also provide a patient with e-mail access to the provider. All of these trends represent potentially disruptive innovations to advance progress.

The rewards will be great for medical practices and hospitals willing to undertake the process of adopting EHRs. These organizations will be well positioned for the future, and some may even create the trends rather than respond to them. Adopters will be well positioned to participate in pay-for-performance initiatives, receiving higher reimbursements and becoming better positioned to comply with federal mandates.

The EHR market remains confusing; however, this book is specifically designed to help you through this journey. The book is organized by sequencing the stages and phases of this journey. It covers the current state of the market and explores the complete optimizing and enhancing of the EHR experience. Proven tools, tips, and strategies are incorporated, and field-tested examples of critical success factors are provided throughout.

SUMMARY

In developing your own EHR history, it is important to know that all great products and services go through stages of evolution and they improve through the process of trial and error. Some people may compare the EHR industry to the banking industry, explaining how you can go anywhere in the world and use an ATM. If only if could be that easy. Unfortunately, healthcare is much more complex—and unlike the banking industry, patients' lives depend on the accuracy of data. ATMs are not known to kill people. Something as enormous and complex as automating healthcare will take considerable time. Consider Woody Allen's statement:

> "If you're not failing every now and again,
> it's a sign you're not doing anything very innovative."[3]

To put this into perspective, in 1958, RCA produced the first eight-track tape for playing music; 40 years later, music is downloaded via the internet on devices smaller then a credit card with no moving parts that can hold hours of digital music.

Just as the music industry evolved, health IT is undergoing a similar journey. Table 2 is a summary of this progress:

Health IT is approximately 30 years into its evolution, with EHRs consuming about 20 years of this evolutionary progression. EHRs are showing clear indications of advancing and improving. Some will argue EHRs have been around much longer; in fact, they have when you consider systems like those used by the Veterans Administration and early attempts by larger health system such as Kaiser Permanente to build their

The Early Years 1975 to 1985	Stand-alone PM systems and HIS with limited ability to capture and store clinical information were common.
The Interface Era 1985 to 2000	Stand-alone EHR systems started to appear, but they had to be interfaced with the above stand-alone PM/HIS systems.
The Enterprise Era 2000 to 2005	EHR and PM vendors started to become one. The single vendor solutions movement was finally here.
The Certification Era 2005 to 2010	Vendors were required to meet and conform to functionality standards important to the adoption of EHRs.
The Data Driven Era Going Forward...	Healthcare providers and systems use data from EHRs in a meaningful way and in accordance with compliance standards with the intent of improving patient safety, lowering cost and improving care.

Table 2: Progression of Health IT

own EHR. EHRs referred to herein are considered "off the shelf" systems being sold on the open market to medical practices and hospitals.

Now, the federal government is taking the most significant measures to date to advance the adoption of EHRs. Incentive money is on the table, followed by financial penalties for not adopting. Much of the cost savings estimated within healthcare reform comes from the benefits expected to come from EHRs. Additional reductions in cost come from reducing Medicare reimbursement for those who do not adopt. In the past, putting off an EHR decision was just a personal choice. Now many are asking, "What is the cost of doing nothing?" or "Can we survive without one?"

Healthcare is by far the most complex industry in the world, touching virtually everyone on the planet; you could say our lives depend on it. Progress in automation is going to take time.

You will be VERY disappointed with your EHR if you are looking for a perfect system. EHRs are not perfect, but neither is the paper chart perfect. More refining and improvements are needed, but providers are now starting to see some legitimate success and tangible benefits.

The purpose of this book is to help you prepare for participating in this process and to help you avoid many of the mistakes made by the early adopters.

REFERENCES

1. Healthcare IT News. IT among top topics at AHIMA, MGMA. http://www.healthcareitnews.com/news/it-among-top-topics-ahima-mgma. Accessed January 10, 2011.

2. Lewis Carroll. http://www.alice-in-wonderland.net/books/1chpt6.html. Accessed July 22, 2010.

3. Woody Allen. BrainyQuote.com, Xplore Inc, 2010. http://www.brainyquote.com/quotes/quotes/w/woodyallen121347.html. Accessed July 22, 2010.

CHAPTER 1

Overview of the EHR Market

INTRODUCTION

Selecting an electronic health record (EHR) system is one of the most important decisions a medical practice can make. It can also be one of the most difficult decisions because of the technical complexity involved in such systems, the sheer number of products available in the marketplace (more than 400 vendors at publication) and the fact that most practices have never before had to undergo such massive operational changes. EHR selection can redefine a practice—and be a career-defining (or career-limiting) decision for its administrators.

This chapter provides an overview of the EHR market, including a brief history of the evolution of these systems. A more thorough understanding of the market will help you better align your decisions with future trends.

Throughout the 50-year history of EHRs, the primary objectives have been (1) to eliminate the paper medical record, (2) to create more convenient access to data, and (3) to improve patient safety and outcomes.

It has been said that implementing an EHR system is like taking a journey; there are a lot of unknowns. Earlier in the evolution of EHR systems, there were far more unknowns. Fortunately, since then, much progress has been made.

Understanding the complexities of the market and some basic history is a good starting point for a successful journey.

BRIEF HISTORY

The history of EHRs can be traced back to the 1960s. Much within today's EHR technology is based on the pioneering work of Lawrence L. Weed, MD. Table 1-1 summarizes the history of EHRs.[1]

Medical professionals have been storing healthcare data electronically since the invention of the personal computer (PC). In fact, healthcare as an industry has benefited the most from information technology. On the diagnostic and clinical side, we now have advances such as electrocardiograms, digital radiology and robotic surgery.

Computer technology and electronic innovation are used extensively throughout healthcare—the one notable exception being the routine management of patient medical records. This "digital divide" is especially true with regard to an ambulatory medical

Time Period	Key Players	Event	Description
1960s	Lawrence L. Weed, MD	Concept Introduced	Weed described a system to automate and reorganize patient medical records to enhance their utilization and thereby lead to improved patient care.
1967	U of VT Team	PROMIS Project	Collaborative effort between physicians and IT experts started at University of Vermont, based on Weed's work. Project objectives: • Develop a system to provide timely and sequential patient data to physician • Enable rapid collection of data for epidemiological studies, medical audits and business audits
Late 1960s	U of VT Team	Development of POMR	Group's efforts produced problem-oriented medical record.
1960s	Mayo Clinic	EHR Development	Mayo began developing electronic medical record systems.

1970		First-time Use	Problem-oriented medical record used in medical ward of Medical Center Hospital of VT
			• Touch-screen technology incorporated into data-entry procedures
			• Drug information elements added to the core program, allowing physicians to check for:
			  – drug actions
			  – dosages
			  – side effects
			  – allergies
			  – interactions
			• Diagnostic and treatment plans devised for 600+ common medical problems

Table 1-1. Time Line for Development of Electronic Health Records (EHRs)

Time Period	Key Players	Event	Description
1970–1980s	Various academic and research institutions	EHRs developed and refined	Period of development and refinement of EMRs: • Technicon system – hospital based • Harvard's COSTAR system – ambulatory care • HELP system – in-patient care • Duke's "The Medical Record" – in-patient care • Indiana's Regenstrief record – combined in-patient care and outpatient care
1990s		Advancements in computer and diagnostic applications	Increase in complexity and more widely used by practices
21st century		Use expands	More and more practices implement EHRs

Adapted from: Pinkerton K. History of electronic medical records. Available at http://EzineArticles.com/?History-Of-Electronic-Medical-Records&id=254240. Accessed January 3, 2011.

Table 1-1. *(Continued)*

practice, which lags behind other forms of medical practice in making the transition. It is often joked that when a FedEx delivery person enters a physician's office, the building's technology infrastructure increases by 200 percent. Even pizza establishments have implemented electronic data systems that can recall stored information such as a caller's street address, previous orders, and preferences (e.g., extra cheese, "hold the sauce"). Unfortunately, healthcare providers still store most patient medical data on paper. When such data is stored electronically, however, it is most often on fragmented and disparate systems that cannot communicate with one another.

When staff files a sheet of paper in a paper medical record, few consider how the paper was originally generated—the actual source. Ninety percent of the time, that piece of paper was originally generated using a PC. Yet, we continue to turn electronic documents into paper that then require manual management. For example, after a patient examination, most physicians dictate their notes on a digital recorder. After the sound file is picked up electronically by a digital transcription system, an electronic document is produced via PC, and the file is saved on a hard drive. Now (this is the insane part), we then take this electronic document and print it out for storage in a paper medical record file folder as a hard copy for 21 years. The fun really begins when that printout goes missing. On occasion, an entire practice will be effectively shut down to locate a missing file.

Rarely does anyone consider the true cost of dealing with paper. Suppose that an EHR vendor offers a system for free—but the catch is that the practice is required to pay the vendor $5.00 each time a new patient record is created in the system. Would you purchase that system? I suspect your answer would be a resounding "No," as you toss the vendor out of the office. Yet, creating a new paper medical record for each new patient *is* paying $5.00 per patient. By the time you add supply costs, inserts, and staff time to assemble and label a new patient paper medical record, the actual cost for these materials ranges from $3.00 to $5.00 per patient. Sometimes it is easy to overlook the costs of paper because we are in the habit of...well, just doing things the only way we know how to do them. Therefore, an important question to begin asking might be, "What is the cost of doing nothing?" (Chapter 9 addresses the concept of return on investment and will help your practice answer this question.)

It may surprise many to know that physicians typically generate only four sheets of paper per patient examination: (1) physician notes, (2) a charge ticket, (3) physician orders, and (4) prescriptions. Although this number can vary by specialty, the main point is that physicians are not causing "the paper problem." Generally, it all comes from the outside—and by the truckload. Healthcare is so regulated, and the concern over proper documentation is so high, that we tend to overkill this process and, in some cases, send duplicates. Consider, for example, how many duplicates of the patient information sheet are sent from the hospital for an admission?

To address this challenge in the late 1970s, vendors started developing solutions that would allow for electronic storage and retrieval of clinical information, creating more convenient access to medical data. EHR vendors have continued to evolve and improve this process since then. Table 1-2 summarizes the past 40 years of this evolution.

During these system evolutions, access methods have also evolved. In the beginning, most systems ran on large mainframe computers with emulating screen images that looked like first-generation video games.

Most early EHR systems were built on-site and remote networking tools were not yet available. Later, dial-up functionality was added via modems and point-to-point T1 lines—both of which were expensive and unreliable. These lines used the existing public infrastructure, making it difficult to obtain reliable bandwidth. Bandwidth, which is usually measured in bits and megabytes, determines how much data can travel across a line and at what speed. Figure 1-1 is an illustration of a modem-connected network.

More recently, virtual private networks (VPN) and multiprotocol label switching networks have leveraged the Internet as a means of connecting multiple computers. Through these networks, physicians can access EHRs from any location with an Internet connection. VPNs are less expensive and more reliable than modem-dependent networks because data is routed using Internet protocol addresses across many different networks through a private tunnel that is only dedicated to your practice. An *Internet protocol address* is a unique code that is assigned to each computer accessing the Internet. This code allows data to travel across many different networks and switches, which creates greater redundancy and less points of failure. Figure 1-2 is an illustration of a VPN.

As for accessing EHR data in the future, most experts predict that cloud computing or software as a service (SaaS) will be the most common access method. *Cloud comput-*

Time Period	Solutions	Technology Type
1970s	Limited, single-purpose repositories. Databases provided only one function (e.g., storing basic demographic information, medications, limited clinical data). The U.S. military was the most advanced with EHRs at this time.	DOS, UNIX, Cobalt, MUMPS Punch card for practice management
1980s	Transaction and financial-management systems. Vendors like IDX, Medical Manager and Medic were supplying this technology. Early versions of stand-alone EHRs were available in the late 1980s.	DOS, UNIX
1990s	Stand-alone EHRs interfaced with stand-alone practice-management systems. These EHRs were basic in functionality and limited in content.	Windows, Linux
2000s	Single vendor, fully integrated solutions operating on a unified platform/database. Most of these solutions were 100 percent Windows-based and many operated exclusively over the World Wide Web. Terms like *application service providers* and *software as a service* (SaaS) started to appear in the marketplace.	Windows, Apple/MAC, .NET programming, Web-based/-enabled
2010s	Subscription-based technologies. Cloud computing and SaaS solutions are expected to become the method of choice for accessing EHR technology.	iPad, mobile devices, cloud computing

Table 1-2: Evolution of Storing and Retrieving Clinical Information Electronically

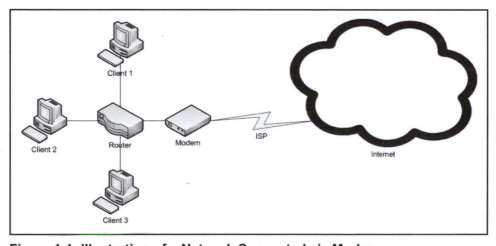

Figure 1-1: Illustration of a Network Connected via Modem

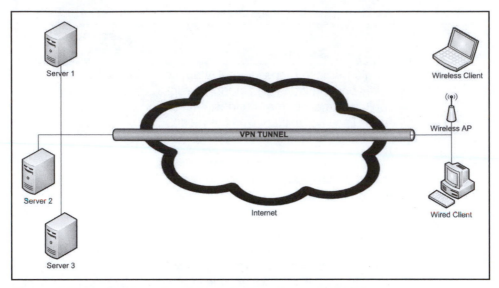

Figure 1-2: Illustration of a Virtual Private Network (VPN)

ing is a metaphor for exclusively using the Internet for all your computing needs. This technology is already widely adopted among social networking sites and virtual companies. In addition, companies like salesforce.com and applications for the iPad are 100 percent virtual, meaning they do not operate on a local hard drive or server. Most of us, by now, have already seen this shift in how we access entertainment, such as movies, books and music. Several EHR vendors are already in the process of converting their systems to SaaS solutions. In fact, many experts predict that physicians will not purchase technology in the future; instead, practices will subscribe to technology, much as we do for basic utilities. Because technology changes so rapidly, SaaS or cloud computing is seen as a much more economical way to deliver and manage electronic systems for a large and geographically dispersed population of users. The only requirements for such systems are an Internet connection and a basic PC. Figure 1-3 is an illustration of SaaS or cloud computing.

Clearly, methods for accessing data have improved dramatically through the years, and, like most technology, the available options have become faster, more reliable and less expensive.

As noted previously, a primary objective of moving to EHRs has always been the improvement of patient safety and outcomes. In 1999, the Institute of Medicine's Committee on the Quality of Healthcare in America released its first report, "Crossing the Quality Chasm: A New Health System for the 21st Century." Researchers found that as many as 98,000 Americans could die each year as a result of a medical errors.[2] Although this report led to a better understanding of patient safety and evidence-based medicine, it did not trigger immediate change. The United States continues to suffer the distinction of being globally recognized for providing high-priced, less-than-optimal healthcare services. The primary barrier to low-cost, high-quality healthcare delivery in the United States is our lack of ability to share and exchange patient data with all caregivers, physician practices, hospitals and payers. However, successful regional efforts

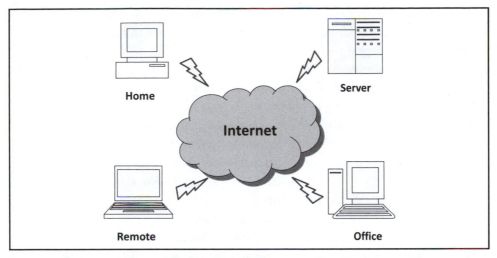

Figure 1-3: Illustration of Software as a Service (SaaS) or Cloud Computing

have been made to address this state of affairs, including immunization repositories and community/regional health information networks.

Although these data-sharing networks offer providers the ability to share and exchange data, most initiatives of this kind have not be successful because there is no economic model to sustain them. Furthermore, regulatory policies, such as the Health Insurance Portability and Accountability Act (HIPAA), create significant barriers to sharing and exchanging health information. The lack of a national identification system is another barrier to system-wide change. Because patient data can be entered into electronic systems in a variety of ways, the same patient may have several different variations of how they are identified within a single system. Consider how many times you have discovered duplicate patient records stored in your practice management system. Now consider how many different practices are treating the same patient. What are the odds that every location enters the patient's information the exact same way?

Healthcare has also been very good at propagating inaccurate patient information. Let's say a patient arrives in the emergency department and the hospital enters his or her information incorrectly. The incorrect information is then spread to the radiologist and treating physician. The patient is later admitted and the incorrect information is passed along to the attending physician who brings the patient's information sheet back to his or her practice the next day for registration and billing. One "minor" data-entry mistake during hospital admission has now been passed along to several caregivers. The practice later catches the mistake and corrects it in their system—but the hospital continues to keep the incorrect information on file. As a result, it is now difficult to exchange information among caregivers because each system identifies the patient differently.

To address this challenge, the government has created the Nationwide Health Information Network (NHIN), which is a set of standards, services and policies that enable secure exchange of health information via the Internet. This network will provide a foundation for the exchange of health information technology (IT) across diverse entities, within communities and across the country—helping to achieve the goals of the

Health Information Technology for Economic and Clinical Health Act. These policies will be replicated across the United States within regional health information exchanges (HIEs). Each HIE will report to the NHIN and all will conform to a common structure for capturing and storing patient data.

The NHIN-HIE initiative is similar to processes in place for the banking industry, which relies on an "interbanking network." Regardless of where your personal financial accounts are held, all banks conform to a single set of standards for transferring and exchanging money (data). In brief, the automated teller machine card you use can be read at every bank around the world. This interoperability allows banks to function without data conflicts. Presently, the federal government is providing millions of dollars to establish nationwide interoperability for the exchange of health information.

Now that we have covered the history, let's address where we are today. On February 24, 2009, President Barack Obama made his first State of the Union address in which he formally announced plans to make a significant investment in EHR technology:

> Our recovery plan will invest in electronic health records and new technology that will reduce errors, bring down costs, ensure privacy, and save lives. It will launch a new effort to conquer a disease that has touched the life of nearly every American...by seeking a cure for cancer in our time. And it makes the largest investment ever in preventive care, because that is one of the best ways to keep our people healthy and our costs under control.[3]

Just prior to this address, the 111th U.S. Congress passed the American Recovery and Reinvestment Act of 2009 (ARRA). The President signed it into law on February 17, 2009. The "stimulus package" was intended to create jobs and promote investment and consumer spending during the recession. The act consisted of $787 billion in spending on a variety of programs and initiatives. Of the $787 billion, $87 billion was devoted to improving healthcare with nearly $26 billion specifically directed toward the promotion of healthcare technology (see Figure 1-4).[4]

Since the passage of ARRA, physicians and hospitals have anxiously awaited further guidance regarding the definition of Meaningful Use for EHRs that will be key to the receipt of financial incentives established under the act for providers who adopt this technology in the time specified (these incentives will be discussed in more detail in Chapter 5). The passage of the new law has become a game-changer in the market because the government is going to start reducing Medicare compensation for physicians who do not adopt a certified system at the conclusion of the EHR incentive program. As a result, EHRs are now a top priority for acute and ambulatory care organizations. Selecting an EHR vendor will be one of the initiatives taken on by hospitals and physician practices across the United States.

Physicians and vendors must become proactive in monitoring EHR technology and legal developments and in considering plans for implementation once ARRA definitions are finalized. The incentives are "time stamped," meaning that late adopters will receive less compensation for implementing these services.

As a result of ARRA's EHR incentives, the market is exploding with vendor options and solutions. Health systems and physicians that were previously "on the fence" about

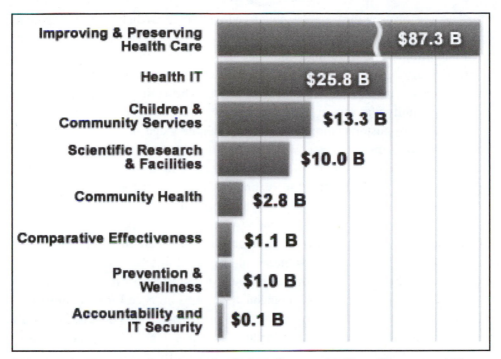

Figure 1-4: Where Your Money Is Going. Source: HHS.gov/Recovery. Where your money is going. http://www.hhs.gov/recovery/. June 10, 2010. Accessed December 22, 2010.

EHRs are now starting to understand the unintentional consequences of not adopting these systems—or being too late to adopt. Thus, the opportunity to participate in ARRA incentive payments and to avoid future penalties drives most of the current interest in EHRs.

Simultaneously, vendors are preparing their products to meet certification requirements. Some are even offering money-back stimulus guarantees. Many vendors face the challenge of redeveloping their old technology to meet the new requirements—or starting from scratch. Several have opted to merge with larger, more established vendors as a way to centralize resources and combine their expertise. One concern among many experts is dealing with practices that adopted earlier versions of EHRs that will not meet the new standards. There are also several "homegrown" solutions that have been developed by individuals on behalf of physicians that will, unfortunately, likely become obsolete. These practices will be faced with the dilemma of converting their old EHR systems over to one that would be incentive eligible. It is also anticipated that many vendors, especially those that have undergone mergers and acquisitions, will discontinue support for their older products as they move to more modern platforms. In Chapter 8, we provide recommendations on how to protect your practice from having its current EHR discontinued.

In the past, vendors with large market share and thousands of customers were considered "safe" options for practice adoption because they were thought to be more financially stable. Although this assumption is true to an extent, the market has made a dramatic shift to products that are capable of responding to uncertainty. For example, some of the more established vendors that have been around for years and have sold multiple versions of their software are now faced with a big challenge of getting all of their clients to conform to new compliance standards. EHRs used to be installed locally, on-site. In addition, more often than not, the software was customized to fit the needs of the practice. As a result, one vendor can potentially have multiple variations of its software, uniquely customized and operating around the United States. In the past, practice compatibility was not an issue. In addition, vendors generally enjoyed additional revenue from customization. However, in this new age of federal compliance and standards, long-time vendors now have to figure out how best to update multiple versions of their software to conform with federal requirements, incorporate the latest cutting-edge technology and retain the customized features customers have come to expect and love. This balancing act is extremely difficult to reach.

Fortunately, Web-based solutions allow vendors to make a single update from a centralized data center. The update is then available to every client instantaneously. This level of functionality is similar to how the social media site Facebook manages its technology. When Facebook makes a simple change to the site, each site subscriber's settings are modified and improved instantaneously. There is no need for Facebook to try to update the personal "page" of each unique customer; the system is operated centrally via the Internet and everyone is subscribing to the service. In addition, although Facebook allows subscribers to customize certain elements on their own pages, individual pages and the entire site conform to the same basic set of standards for all users.

Vendors have taken notice. The concept of online software distribution has taken off. It is seen as the best way to keep down costs, improve vendor accessibility, and speed up vendor response to evolving compliance standards. Many larger vendors have already started to develop Web-based solutions and have begun acquiring companies. As a result, experts expect to see an explosion of Internet-based solutions, or cloud-based computing, emerging in the market in the next few years.

In addition, the market is also flooded with niche-based, healthcare-specific technology companies. These niche-based solutions are even offered by large, national corporations like AT&T, Google Inc., IBM Corporation and Microsoft Corporation. Because of the popularity of EHRs and the $20 billion in federal stimulus money offered, many companies started looking for ways to "cash in" on the new market. Some examples of niche products include personal health records, electronic prescribing, handheld charge capturing, patient portals, content providers, and transaction companies (e.g., electronic data exchange vendors). Most niche vendors are promoting their solution as a way to enhance existing EHR systems—a new level of customization and functionality. In some cases, major EHR vendors resell these niche solutions under a private label or as a distributor on behalf of the niche company.

Healthcare IT News recently published an article on this topic that describes how the market has a significant trail of solutions that are being carried by the larger vendors and how smaller, niche vendors exist among them.[5] Smaller vendors are more nimble and are not weighted down with older systems to support. In most cases, niche vendors are running on Web-based solutions that give them even greater leverage in a market that expects vendors to turn on a dime to meet compliance standards. The article continues:

Physicians are not a homogeneous group of customers and it is very unlikely that that the utilitarian large EMR vendors will be able to satisfy the majority of the market. Multiple niche opportunities already exist in providing services tailored to particular medical specialties and various practice models, such as medical homes, concierge medicine, telemedicine, micro practices and more.[5]

The article goes on to say:

More niche opportunities will be created by physician work-flow preferences and proliferation of non-physician providers. Tail companies that learn how to answer the needs of these niches by providing high quality solutions, while keeping the costs of customization and service to a minimum, will thrive.[5]

CONCLUSION

The EHR market has certainly evolved significantly during the past several years, much like we have gone from eight-track tape players to MP3 players. Although there has been a lot of trial and error, most of the evolutionary change in EHRs is seen as a "net positive" and further improvements are being made every day. Adoption levels are still low, but there are some significant federal financial incentives being offered to help physicians make the change. Some financial penalties will come in the future for practices that choose not to adopt EHRs. It is also understood that late adopters will not receive as much ARRA stimulus funding as others and will be confronted with potential reductions to Medicare reimbursement.

As for the evolution of EHRs, product functionality and access to data have been the most improved features. As more physicians use EHRs, the market benefits from their knowledge and feedback.

Now, the Internet is seen as the primary tool for accessing, connecting and exchanging EHR information. A lot of work still has to be done to ensure patient privacy. In addition, there is a need to standardize the way we record and store data. However, basic connectivity is now very affordable and reliable. There are also multiple options for accessing the Internet, and it is common to find a connection anywhere business is being conducted.

Patient safety, cost containment and improved clinical outcomes are driving this change from the government's perspective. These factors are also the primary impetus for ARRA stimulus incentives. Compliance standards are a way to ensure that the overall system benefits from ARRA stimulus dollars and that, in the long run, the revised system is actually saving tax-payer money. Creating HIE standards is the first step in the process and will be a significant undertaking during the next several years.

As for the vendors, we expect to see more mergers and some discontinuation of older EHR systems as vendors meet new compliance standards. Disruptive technology vendors (e.g., niche vendors), major corporations aligning with EHRs, SaaS providers, and solutions that operate on iPads are all making their way into the marketplace. The impact of these upcoming changes remains unknown. However, looking back at the past is a good way to predict the future, and the past clearly shows that health IT will continue to evolve and improve.

REFERENCES

1. Pinkerton K. History of electronic medical records. http://ezinearticles.com/?expert=Kent_Pinkerton Accessed January 3, 2011.

2. Institute of Medicine. *To Err is Human: Building a Safer Health System.* Washington, DC: National Academies Press; 1999.

3. President Barack Obama's State of the Union Address. February 24, 2009. Available at http://www.whitehouse.gov/the_press_office/Remarks-of-President-Barack-Obama-Address-to-Joint-Session-of-Congress/. Accessed January 10, 2011.

4. HHS.gov/Recovery. Where your money is going. http://www.hhs.gov/recovery/. June 10, 2010. Accessed December 22, 2010.

5. Gur-Arie M. The long tail of the EMR. *Healthcare IT News.* October 9, 2009. http://www.healthcareitnews.com/blog/long-tail-emr. Accessed August 18, 2010.

CHAPTER 2

EHR Critical Success Factors

INTRODUCTION

Successful use of electronic health records (EHRs) requires defining the organizational goals that will be fulfilled by their use, selecting a vendor with values and goals that are congruent with practice goals, and planning for the implementation, ongoing management and development of the EHR system. Long-term success with EHRs is dependent on establishing a continuous process of assimilating the features and functionality of this technology into the fabric of the practice.

Critical success factors are the elements necessary to accomplish a specified goal. Critical success factors for EHRs include:

- Change management
- Completion of a readiness assessment
- Buy-in and contribution from stakeholders, including physicians
- Ability to report on evaluation metrics established for each phase of the project
- Training before, during, and after EHR implementation
- How leadership deals with technology malfunctions

Operationally, the critical success factors medical practice leadership needs to consider are the following:

- A governance plan that ensures uniform adoption and assimilation of the system.
- Reliable information technology (IT) infrastructure.
- A well-designed system that supports practice workflow and workload.
- A deliberate implementation plan that capitalizes on the strengths of the clinic or health center and minimizes its weaknesses.
- Standardized workflow and processes, as established through a collaborative effort among administration, providers, and staff.
- Ongoing management and development that ensures optimal use of EHRs.

Physician groups, both private and hospital-owned groups, decide they are ready for EHR technology for many reasons. A significant driver is the government mandate and tax incentives to use EHRs. Although many groups will not meet the 2012 deadline for maximum stimulus participation, most groups do not want to be left behind when there are penalties for not using EHRs. A decision based purely on tax incentives, how-ever, frequently does not lead to positive, successful assimilation of this technology.

Other drivers can include:

- Improved quality of care, documentation, staff efficiency and patient safety.
- Decreased medical errors and healthcare delivery costs.
- Improved revenue and a compressed revenue cycle.
- Increased staff interest in improved access and management of clinical data.

EHRs improve the quality of care by providing decision support at the point of patient contact. In the case of chronic illness, built-in triggers prompt physicians to order tests that could prevent disease progression and improve patient health. In the case of preventive care, patient protocols can be built in (or downloaded) to encourage providers to order preventive screening or provide counseling that improves overall health within a specified patient population. In the case of acute illness, EHRs can sug-gest treatment options.

Many groups experience improved efficiency when they adopt and assimilate EHRs. They find that EHRs are capable of putting the right information in front of the right person at the right time. EHRs also allow patient requests to be handled by fewer people and satisfied more quickly. This process, in turn, leads to fewer phone calls and steps to follow up on simple requests, such as obtaining copies of medical records or prescrip-tion refills. It also leads to better utilization of highly trained (and paid) provider staff. For example, a patient calling in for an appointment can be told that getting labora-tory work performed one week prior to an office visit will allow the provider to review test results in person with the patient. Furthermore, with EHRs there are no more lost medical records—and many fewer steps to get the results of laboratory and radiology studies back to the provider and entered in the patient's medical record.

In most cases, a provider can "template" a visit and—using a point-and-click method—document findings, "tee up" follow-up studies for tracking, pass charges to the billing system, and, in most cases, ensure that he/she is providing the "gold stan-dard" of care to every patient, every time. That said, EHRs will improve efficiency only if they are properly deployed and supported.

Through the use of decision-support applications and drug-to-drug and drug-to-allergy testing, EHRs help providers improve patient safety and decrease medication errors. Most EHR systems use an external database to support prescribing practices. These databases present the provider with dosing options and may even suggest a lower cost alternative. In addition, when medications are added as discreet data, they can be cross-checked within the patient's medical history to ensure that (1) he/she will not have an adverse reaction, and (2) the drug is not already a part of his/her prescribed medication regimen.

Managing paper medical records is expensive. It requires a tremendous amount of staff to manage paper systems properly. Paper records are easily misplaced (or even lost), and basic data-entry tasks require many hands and many steps. Also, paper records are available to only one person at a time.

Although the up-front costs of EHR technology are significant (i.e., approximately $55,000 per provider for installation, deployment, and implementation), its cost over time is significantly less than managing paper. For example, EHRs decrease wasteful spending on diagnostic tests by eliminating duplicate testing and helping to ensure that the correct tests are ordered for any given illness. EHRs also help the bottom line by compressing the revenue cycle. In most cases, visit charges can be sent on the day of service.

Providers continuously struggle to provide documentation that is individualized, complete and comprehensive, and, most importantly, describes what happened at the office visit for the next person reading the documentation. EHRs help providers document and place orders. In paper medical records, information frequently must be written in several places, which guarantees that it will *not* appear in at least one of those places. However, many providers and certified coders struggle with the lack of individuality allowed in EHR office notes. For the best results, providers should use the point-and-click method provided by templates, augmenting standard EHR documentation to provide the level of individuality necessary for the patient.

Most importantly, EHRs provide access to a large volume of clinical data that is simply not possible with paper records. Although computers are not very good at critical thinking or applying clinical judgment, they are excellent at storing, remembering, retrieving and presenting data in a format that can be easily analyzed. Provider analysis will lead to improved quality of care for many diseases and illnesses.

GOVERNANCE

Decisive and clear governance is a critical success factor in EHR adoption and assimilation. It is essential to create the staff infrastructure that will allow for the successful completion of a project of this complexity. The governance team provides a steady infusion of motivation and leadership, as well as an awareness of practice culture that ensures the inclusion of stakeholders and wise information management (e.g., setting expectations).

In this setting, *motivation* consists of the persuasion, incentive and inducement necessary to assimilate EHR technology within the practice. During EHR implementation, motivation can come in many forms, such as educating clinical staff on the features and functionality of the system (persuasion). It can also involve establishing evaluation metrics and looking for opportunities to offer small rewards to staff for meeting or exceeding goals (incentive). For example, one might establish the number of medical records each staff member is expected to manually enter, or *preload*, in a given period and then reward individuals when they meet (or exceed) that goal with a modest department store gift card.

Motivation can also take the form of a stick. Although persuasion and incentive are certainly preferable to inducement, practice staff must understand that using EHRs is a requirement of employment. Similarly, physician staff must understand that using EHRs is not optional.

The first step in establishing good governance for an EHR project is to identify a physician champion within the practice. This physician advocate plays a critical role of transformational leadership and should be respected for his/her comfort with and knowledge of IT as well as his/her knowledge and understanding of practice culture. That said, choosing an early adopter of EHR technology may not be the best choice in a physician champion. It is often best to focus on enlisting a medical leader who is well respected, has a good understanding of practice culture, works collaboratively with top-level leadership, can influence broad groups of peers and demonstrates good IT understanding and use. The physician champion should also be viewed as an advocate by his/her associates. This respected proponent should view the role of technology in healthcare not as a panacea that will solve all problems, but, rather, as a tool that can improve the efficiency, effectiveness and safety of patient care.

In addition, top management has an important role to play in EHR implementation projects. Chiefly, they must demonstrate an unwavering commitment to the success of the project as well as an awareness of the capabilities and limitations of EHRs. They must work in collaboration with the physician leader and practice administrators to create reasonable, attainable goals for the project, staff and physicians. Top management and the physician leader must also be able to communicate IT strategy to all employees and exhibit a strong commitment to incorporating IT. Leaders must exhibit resolve by holding project managers accountable to performance standards, such as meeting project milestones. In addition, the training provided should allow staff and physicians to have a sense of competence and confidence when using the system. EHR projects most often fail when they are handed off from top-level leadership to technical experts.

Practice culture is a crucial determinant of how EHRs need to be implemented in a practice. A young, progressive practice will likely move more quickly and be more tolerant of technology malfunctions than an older, more traditional practice. It is important to understand that many older physicians have been interacting with paper medical records in a particular way for 20 to 30 years. Transitioning to EHRs can be difficult in this setting. When there is resistance to change, the transition will be that much more difficult, time consuming and expensive.

EHR implementation projects are fraught with uncertainty. Although project managers and the implementation team try to account for every possible scenario, it is nearly impossible to account for everything.

The antidote to uncertainty is good communication. The governance team must control the content and flow of information related to the project. Adopting a communication plan that addresses project milestones, staff requirements and project vision is a key to success.

The communication plan should be organized by those who will develop message content (i.e., at least one member of the governance team) and those who will help determine what, when and how (e.g., posters, e-mail, company intranet messages) the information will be disseminated. The plan needs to address how the practice will communicate with patients and with associated healthcare providers in the community. Many practice groups communicate with patients using posters in waiting and examination areas as well as messages on practice statements.

Choosing a theme and name for the EHR project is another effective communication tool. The theme can be incorporated into staff incentive programs and help create a lighter atmosphere as the practice comes closer to launching the system. Humor and whimsy go a long way toward lowering staff anxiety and improving morale as the final transition to a live EHR environment becomes imminent.

Inclusion of the stakeholders is essential to the success of any EHR project, and the governance team is responsible for ensuring these individuals are included at key phases of the project. In almost all decisions related to the EHR, it is important to include key physicians, technology staff, nursing or medical assistant staff, as well as staff from medical records, billing/coding and risk management. The opportunity for success is improved by asking stakeholders to work with the implementation team to (1) run workflows in the context of the new system, (2) test clinical content, and (3) regularly communicate their expectations regarding project functionality.

IT INFRASTRUCTURE

Most groups will need to upgrade their IT infrastructure when implementing EHR technology. IT infrastructure must be robust and reliable, with fast and reliable networking, enough of the correct end-user hardware, proper housing for server hardware and adequate help desk support.

When selecting a system, practice groups will need to choose between a client-server model software or a software as a service (SaaS) model. Typically, larger, more complex practice groups choose client-server systems and SaaS model software is preferred by smaller groups.

A client-server system requires a robust and reliable local area network that allows local computers, printers and scanners to connect to the application and the database where patient data are stored. In many cases, Internet access is required to allow multiple sites to connect to each other and to the application and database servers. Internet access must be high speed and dedicated to the EHR system. In addition, it is important to consider redundancy in the event that the primary Internet connection goes down or is not available.

SaaS models are completely reliant on a robust, reliable Internet connection because the practice will be accessing a system that is housed off site. In this case, the application and database are housed at the vendor's data center and, although all data are owned by the practice, there is a subscription fee associated with the use of software licenses and database access. Redundant Internet connection is a requirement for practices using an SaaS model. In either model, creating a network that maximizes broadband speed to each workstation and works easily and reliably is a critical success factor.

End-User Access Models and Peripherals

How end-users (i.e., providers and staff) access EHRs is another part of the IT infrastructure that the governance team must consider. There are two choices: (1) workstations in every examination room and at each provider's and staff member's desk or (2) individual tablet PCs (personal computers) or laptop devices that connect wirelessly.

Although handhelds can be effective tools for viewing some data, such as laboratory and radiology results, such devices generally do not provide enough screen "real estate" to make them effective tools for inputting EHR data. Perhaps for this reason, they are not widely used for EHR systems. In addition, currently, they are not widely supported by the major EHR vendors. However, with the recent introduction of the Apple iPhone and iPad, it is only a matter of time before EHR applications will be supported by vendors for these popular devices.

Outfitting each examination room with a thin-client EHR workstation allows one to create a simple deployment that is relatively inexpensive and easy to maintain. The main disadvantage of this set-up, however, is that it requires each user to log on and off during each patient encounter. Because EHRs house protected health information, a powerful, difficult-to-break password is required. Unfortunately, most providers object to the length and complexity of a *strong password*—preferably auto-generated and typically consisting of eight characters with at least one numeral, a character, and a capital letter—and will not be willing to enter it with every encounter. When using a thin-client EHR system, there is a significant risk that providers or staff will leave workstations running out of convenience or as a result of haste. Soon, patient information will be entered using someone else's username and password, essentially falsifying patient medical records.

Another disadvantage to this deployment model is that it requires supporting more workstations (i.e., one per provider plus one for every examination room). Finally, providers and staff cannot make full use of the features and functionality of most EHR systems in this deployment model. Most wireless-based EHR systems notify providers of patient arrival and readiness to be seen, but this feature is not available in a thin-client environment. Furthermore, other communication methods supported by wireless-based EHR systems (e.g., electronic delivery of laboratory and diagnostic test results, notification of prescription refill requests and notification of patient and other referring/referral provider communication) are not available. When EHRs are available only from examination rooms and at provider and staff members' desks, the just-in-time communication features supported by many EHR systems are limited.

When laptops or tablet PCs are used, a wireless network must be deployed to allow for connection of the devices to the network. Although wireless networks require specialized skills for proper installation and configuration, wireless access points are becoming easier to deploy and manage as they become ubiquitous in medical settings. The advantages of wireless EHR deployments are improved system features and functionality, fewer log-ins, and improved security, including secure user credentials for data entry. This type of deployment requires that each provider and clinic staff member is issued one device, either a laptop or tablet PC. Providers should be permitted to take their devices home or to other clinical locations. This deployment model limits the number of machines/devices that the organization must support.

The main disadvantages of this type of system are mostly related to the level of IT skill required to support and maintain the system and the expense of the devices and wireless connections. Although laptop and tablet PCs are more expensive initially, outfitting providers and staff (rather than rooms) requires fewer machines and, in most cases, the costs are offset.

The remaining infrastructure issues are fax servers, printers, scanners and remote access. A fax server is the most efficient way to manage incoming and outgoing fax messages. Most EHR systems allow faxes to come directly to the desktop of the recipient and allow providers and staff to fax directly from their desktops. Although it is relatively simple to configure outgoing PC-based fax capabilities, enabling incoming faxes generally requires more thought and work, depending on the fax server used. Typically, incoming faxes require workflow considerations and the proper fax equipment to receive the fax. Most new (i.e., less than three years old) computers incorporate fax servers and can handle in-bound faxes.

While the practice is transitioning to an EHR system, there will be an ongoing need to print and handle paper coming into the practice. Mapping printers and using a naming convention for them that is easily understood by staff will minimize printing frustration and support issues. It is also important to consider printer location. Meaningful use guidelines require that the patient receive printed instructions at the end of each visit. These instructions should be printed in the clinical area and delivered by a medical assistant or nurse, allowing the patient one last opportunity to ask questions before leaving the office. Making a printer easily accessible for this purpose improves patient flow.

Scanning is an essential component of any good EHR system. Using dedicated scanners and workstations ensures the highest level of efficiency for the medical records department. Networked scanners are not as efficient because they are typically multi-function machines; a fax or printout can arrive in the middle of the scanning process.

Remote access is essential for the efficient use of EHRs. Providers and others supporting EHRs must be able to access data from locations outside the clinic network. This level of accessibility requires publishing EHR data to a secure website or deploying a virtual provider network, which requires installing a software client on each workstation that will access EHR data remotely. In either case, creating remote access requires specialized IT skills.

SYSTEM DESIGN

System design is a critical success factor for good system adoption and assimilation. A well-designed system supports the workflow and workload of the practice. Ensuring that your practice has a well-designed EHR system begins at the system-selection stage of the process and continues through the implementation phase when the system is customized. Design includes addressing clinical content and other set-up issues, such as messaging features, physician orders, prescription refill management, results management, documentation of communication with patients, and managing clinical documents management.

During the planning process, the practice must examine the workflow and workload of several processes. At a minimum, they need to consider:

- Preloading patient medical records to accommodate the transition to EHRs
- Prescription refills
- Referral requests
- Patient phone calls for issues other than refill and referral requests
- Patient visit flow, including check-in and checkout
- Dictation and transcription
- Laboratory and radiology orders and results
- Patient follow up on diagnostic tests and referral results
- Paper workflow for paper documents still coming into the practice
- Release-of-information requests

Mapping current workflows using a *swim lane diagram* is the first step in re-engineering workflow for the EHR. Swim lane diagrams identify all of the actors in a given process, indicating all of the processes the actor performs and the sequence in which they are performed, along with any hand-offs from one actor to another.

EHR workflow re-engineering is then documented on a separate swim lane diagram. This diagram is used as the foundation for all EHR training materials. After workflows are re-engineered, the EHR team reviews them in the context of the EHR, making sure that all processes are accounted for, that the processes are in the correct sequence and that the hand-offs are accurate. A combination of workflow documentation and training materials ultimately become the policy manual for the organization. Therefore, each document should be developed and organized with this deliverable in mind.

During EHR implementation, it is important to track and monitor workload. Many processes will become more efficient, requiring fewer steps—and, in many cases, fewer people. However, during the implementation phase, the practice must continue the processes necessary to maintain paper medical records, changing existing processes and evaluating the new processes put in place. At times, implementation can be overwhelming to staff. Although it may be tempting to bring on additional staff, it is generally best to hire temporary staff and/or look for opportunities to shift existing staff into critical positions. Re-engineering workflow to standardize and improve efficiency for EHRs can assist in keeping workloads manageable. Furthermore, try to resist maintaining parallel paper and electronic processes whenever possible.

IMPLEMENTATION PLANNING

Implementation planning is a critical success factor. Implementation planning includes considering an overall plan and time line for the project. This plan should include a delineation and assignment of responsibility for all tasks related to each phase of the project. Typically, an EHR project has a "build phase" that includes set-up of server and end-user hardware, loading of software, network design and deployment and security assignments. This phase of the project can take 90 to 120 days, depending on the need for network infrastructure re-design and deployment. Adding bandwidth and converting to fiber optic or multiprotocol label switching networks requires telecom providers to make adjustments and can take 45 to 60 days. These requirements will not be vendor-dependent and should be initiated during the vendor-contracting phase because most EHRs require robust and reliable wide area and local area networking regardless of the vendor selected.

Once the EHR system is installed, critical tables will need to be built. These include:

- Adding users
- Building custom lists
- Establishing a connection from the practice management system for exchanging patient demographic information
- Setting up electronic prescribing (E-prescribing) functionality
- Setting up document management systems
- Loading content and making the necessary customizations

All functionality must be tested before user training and before launching the EHR system for use in the live environment.

Making the transition from paper to an electronic environment requires preloading patient data from paper medical records to EHRs. This phase of implementation gives physicians and staff an opportunity to gain experience navigating in EHRs and helps them begin to understand the logic of the system.

Additional implementation planning involves the components of training. A training methodology must be adopted: direct training from the vendor for all end-users, or a train-the-trainer approach when "super users" or "power users" can be identified. Super users are trained by the vendor before they, in turn, proceed to train an assigned number of end-users within the practice.

A training curriculum for each phase of the project must be developed to ensure that critical functionality is taught to end-users in the proper sequence. After workflow changes are delineated, training materials that reflect adjusted workflows for various processes must be developed.

Each phase should also have documented evaluation metrics, such as the number of preloads each physician and staff member is expected to perform during the course of a week, the number of refills and new prescriptions processed through the E-prescribing feature, accurate placement of physician orders and disposition of laboratory and diagnostic result reports. Unit managers must be trained in how to track and report progress.

CONCLUSION

Creating an awareness of crucial success factors guides the planning and evaluation of a project of this magnitude. Keeping administrators focused on success and using the elements discussed in this chapter improves the opportunity to routinize high-functionality use of EHRs.

CHAPTER 3

Getting Prepared for the EHR Transition— From Paper to Electronic

INTRODUCTION

You are the chief executive officer (CEO) or the executive director of a healthcare practice, and you can see the handwriting on the wall: adopt an electronic health record (EHR) system or risk lagging behind the technology curve...or worse yet, a reduction in Medicare revenue. You are also faced with the opportunity to participate in quality initiatives from insurers, state health departments, and others that could mean real dollars for your bottom line. In today's healthcare market, reporting on quality indicators means increased dollars.

You have also heard the horror stories. Tales include EHR projects that have landed practices at the bank asking for loans to make payroll, physicians who never again achieve their pre-EHR production levels, providers quitting rather than using EHRs and administrators who have lost their jobs secondary to poorly implemented EHRs. You know you have to make the move, but how do you prepare for a success story rather than a horror show?

Chapter 2, EHR Critical Success Factors, presents the areas that need your attention in order to improve the opportunities for success. This chapter discusses how to prepare for managing the transition from paper to electronic. There are a few axioms to keep in mind as you prepare:

- You are not embarking on an information technology (IT) project; you are embarking on a clinical transformation—a change management project.
- Nobody likes change and, to borrow a phrase, you are about to "move the cheese," as well as change the flavor of the cheese and alter the portion size. Do not expect a smooth ride.[1]
- Although providers are very intelligent people, sometimes they are not very good at admitting when they do not know something.
- There is no substitution for leadership and education in an EHR project. There must be strong, confident, unwavering support for the EHR. In addition, every-

one must learn the logic behind the project and practice with the system to become accustomed to navigation in the EHR.

- This too shall pass. Most, if not all, groups using an EHR today went through a storm to get there. That said, even those who weathered tornado-like conditions would not go back to paper.

CLINICAL TRANSFORMATION

The EHR will affect every aspect of the business of a clinical practice. It affects how health information is viewed, managed, tracked, acted on, and communicated to patients. It affects billing practices, coding practices, workload distribution and basic workflow for the entire practice—providers, staff and patients. The first step in preparation is embracing this fact. The second step in preparing for EHRs is looking for the areas where transforming the paper process will provide huge improvements. The third step in this transformation is educating providers and staff on the knowledge, skills and attitudes necessary to transform the practice successfully.

The EHR will affect every aspect of the practice. Viewing health information on a computer screen and flipping through a paper-based medical record are two very different processes. The EHR presents the same information in a number of views (e.g., medical record summary view, document view, report view), it is available for view by multiple people at the same time (e.g., provider, nursing staff, billing) and it provides a "just enough, just-in-time" view of clinical data that improves efficiency, decreases waste, decreases medical error and improves patient safety *if* it is properly configured and these features are embraced.

If EHRs are configured like paper medical records, their functionality is lost and the clinical transformation will be incomplete. Billing and coding staff must embrace the fact that EHRs are intended to provide point-of-care decision support and that they are designed to allow providers to code more accurately. Too often coders would rather code for the provider rather than educate them as to how to code more effectively; it is considered job security.

As administrators prepare for the EHR transformation, they must communicate that the new system will affect everyone and that job security is now dependent on collaboration and embracing the change. Coders will need to be prepared to input clinical content that ensures federal compliance and improves the ability of providers to code at the point of care. One example is modifying descriptors on diagnoses codes to make them more user friendly. Rhinitis, for example, can become "runny nose" in the system as long as the code for rhinitis is associated with the descriptor "runny nose." There is a tendency toward precision and inflexibility on the part of coders that can sometimes hamper the EHR transition.

The EHR will also affect the workflow and workload distribution in the practice. Clinical roles are more defined in the electronic world because security levels need to be assigned to every member of the practice. Workflows must be mapped both in the current state and then in the future state of the EHR. Furthermore, there must be a "design, build, and verify" process associated with workflow engineering. Practice experts (trusted members of the clinical team in the practice) must describe to the EHR experts how a particular process is accomplished in the practice. These experts must pay particular attention to the paper cues that will no longer be in place when the switch is made to the electronic environment. Next, the processes must be redesigned by the EHR experts for the electronic world, visually mapped, and then presented back to the clinical stakeholders in the context of the new system for verification and refinement. Administrators must prepare for the commitment of time needed to complete this process. There is no room for rushing the process.

Providers will take over more of the workload in the electronic environment. Quite simply, in the electronic environment—when the EHR is well designed and properly configured—it is easier for providers to personally perform a process (e.g., prescribe or refill a medication, order a diagnostic test) than it is to tell a staff member to do it. Providers often balk at this new reality, declaring, "I will not become a data-entry clerk." However, providers have been entering data in paper medical records since the beginning of time. Until now though, they have entered this data by recording words into a dictation device, scribbling words on a page or verbally telling a staff person to enter information. In EHRs, only the communication tool has changed; it is a computer rather than a voice or pen. Providers will need to be prepared that communication with staff via computer is the goal and requirement of the new EHR system.

During the period leading up to system selection and implementation, consider the workflow and workload areas within the practice that are less than optimal today. For example, are unlicensed medical assistants refilling medications? Currently, many EHRs do not distinguish security levels for prescription refills only, and granting security for medication management may mean that the medical assistant can now sign all prescriptions, even if only on the behalf of the provider. EHR adoption may be an opportunity to tighten internal processes and not accept risks of an unlicensed staff member abusing the privilege.

In the new EHR environment, patients will have greater access to their own health information. Meaningful Use guidelines require a practice to make health information available to patients in an electronic format (e.g., website or patient portal). Patients will also now have the ability to communicate with providers electronically. Although this new level of accessibility is a clear benefit to patients, many providers have expressed concerns about managing this new level of access with regard to provider workflow and maintaining the privacy of health information. Setting reasonable policies and expectations for this type of communication that is in keeping with the culture of the practice and the community can help providers and staff to become more comfortable. Providers and staff may need to be reminded that a proactive, engaged patient really does improve the experience for both the patient and the provider.

Look for areas within the practice where clinical processes could be improved. A good place to start is the literature coming out of the Institute for Healthcare Improvement (www.ihi.org), HIMSS (www.himss.org), and the Medical Group Management Association (www.mgma.com). Administrators may also wish to attend user group conferences for the EHR vendors under consideration. Although many vendors insist that only contracted users can attend such events, they will (when pressed) generally allow attendance during a practice's EHR system selection process.

Educating staff and providers on clinical transformation, process improvement, and mapping and reengineering workflows prepares them for what is about to come.

The importance of process improvement—and not allowing EHR implementation to become an opportunity to "pave the cow path"—cannot be emphasized enough. A well-known, well-worn, "comfortable" path is not always the most direct, most efficient—or even the safest—way of getting to where you are going. At all steps, the practice must be encouraged to resist the tendency to build the EHR in the image of the paper system it is replacing. As best you can, understand and incorporate the notion that life is about to become very different and the processes will continuously be reviewed and evaluated for efficiency, safety, and improvement to the revenue bottom line and patient and provider experiences.

The EHR will transform the clinical practice "by hook or by crook." Attitudes toward this transformation can make the process either easier or harder. Let the staff know early on in the project that clinical transformation is the expectation and goal. Start examining clinical processes quickly after the decision to move to EHRs is made. Commit the proper resources to clinical process review and workflow reengineering in preparation for this change.

CHANGE MANAGEMENT

In preparation for the intense change management that will be central to this transformation from paper to electronic, leaders must understand and appreciate the history of a practice, its organizational structure, and the culture of the practice as well as the community it serves. In addition, leaders must understand how the people (providers, staff, and patients) function within this culture. This is the sociology of change. Embracing this approach improves the practice's potential for successful transformation.

Organizational culture is comprised of the assumptions, values, norms, and tangible artifacts of the organization or practice. Indications of an organizational culture are events that occur, or things people talk about or want to show off. It is the elements that would give you clues as to an individual's personality. What do they value? What is important to them? How do they present themselves to the community, including patients?

It is useful to consider the competing values approach when analyzing organizational culture. Although each practice displays certain elements of each cultural "type," there is usually evidence that a practice favors one type over another. Table 3-1 describes the three main organizational culture types using the competing values approach to understanding clinical culture.

Most experts agree that a strong understanding of a practice's cultural environment and, more importantly, the strengths and weaknesses of that environment will assist groups in staying current and making change easier to manage. Successful change or transition management comes through awareness: awareness of culture; awareness of what EHRs can and cannot do; awareness that the new system will affect every aspect of the practice; and awareness of how difficult change can be for many people, especially those who are highly competent, confident and comfortable in their current roles. The key is to develop awareness of organizational culture and effectively manage it in such a way that the group can capitalize on strengths and mitigate weaknesses, create synergy and effectively weather conflict.

Cultural Type	Description	Example
Consensual or clan culture	**Organizational focus:** people **Leadership style:** mentoring, parenting **Employee management:** teamwork, participation, loyalty **Organizational glue:** loyalty, trust **Strategic emphasis:** human development **Criteria for success:** development of human resources, teamwork, concern for people	Independent practices, particularly those that have grown through acquisition of other, smaller practices
"Ad hoc-racy"	**Organizational focus:** entrepreneurial, risk taking **Leadership style:** innovative **Employee management:** innovative, freedom, uniqueness **Organizational glue:** commitment to innovation, development **Strategic emphasis:** acquisition of resources, creating new challenges **Criteria for success:** unique and new products and services	Intensive care units, emergency departments, surgery, some independent practices
Hierarchy	**Organizational focus:** control, structure **Leadership style:** coordinating, organized, oriented toward efficiency **Employee management:** security, conformity, predictability **Organizational glue:** formal rules, policies **Strategic emphasis:** permanence, stability **Criteria for success:** dependable, efficient, low cost	Government-provided healthcare, federally qualified health centers, critical access, veterans organizations, hospital-owned practices

Table 3-1: Competing Values Approach to Describing Organizational Culture

One of the roles of organizational culture is to assist the group in balancing competing technical needs. Cultural orientation includes ways of thinking and behaving with respect to change, diversity, conflict, innovation, organizational learning, knowledge management, partnership or alliance building, relationship formation and corporate responsibility. Because a majority of physicians practice in settings with fewer than 10 providers, implementing EHRs has been difficult. In fact, even in large multispecialty groups, most providers function within a department or unit of no more than 10 providers. The prevailing culture in such a setting is generally the "clan," which focuses on individual growth and development rather than that of the organization as whole. In fact, most physicians practicing in this sort of environment struggle to understand why EHRs are necessary at all because, to their way of thinking, "Everything is just fine as it is." Although this is a pretty straightforward concept, the devil is in the details. Awareness is the first step.

Developing cultural awareness comes through:

- Strategic planning.
- Using the awareness derived from strategic planning to ensure that consistency threads through organizational mission, goals, strategies, structures, and processes.
- Understanding that the deliverable from strategic planning and the ensuing awareness is the development of formal statements of organizational philosophy and values that are communicated to staff and patients.

Strategic planning sessions in preparation for EHR adoption improve everyone's understanding of the goals, objectives, and expectations for the new system.

Schein identified several essential elements for organizational success. These elements parallel those of successful implementation projects. Table 3-2 provides a comparison of these elements. Although each of these essential elements is important, the underpinnings of a strong cultural foundation (values, behavioral norms and patterns, and symbols) provide the necessary reinforcement.

The first step in any change process is the application of "heat" to "unfreeze" the current situation. In this context, "heat" is a problem, an opportunity, a changed circumstance, and/or accumulated excesses or deficiencies. For example, two problems with paper medical records are that they are expensive and often go missing. A group that is consistently frustrated by seeing patients with incomplete medical records can redirect that frustration and use it as a motivation to change the status quo and make the leap to EHRs.

It is true that the American Recovery and Reinvestment Act of 2009 (ARRA) is an opportunity for providers to receive financial assistance with the cost of adopting EHRs. However, in the meantime, the need to comply with government regulatory standards for quality is a changed circumstance. The fact that Medicare reimbursements will soon be lowered for practices not using EHRs in a "meaningful" way is a sufficient motivator for most providers and practices to make the change. The problem is that this latter form of motivation is a "stick" rather than a "carrot." People generally respond better when they are not forced into changes. As leadership prepares for this transition, it may be useful to downplay ARRA as a reason or motivation and reframe the act as a tool that will make the assimilation of EHRs possible. In turn, EHRs make

Elements for EHR Success	
Successful Implementation	**Successful Organizations**
Clearly articulates organizational requirements to the vendor; does not allow a "one-size-fits-most," drive-by implementation.	Proactive, not reactive
Accepts that implementation and go-live are just the beginning, not the end. Commits adequate resources. The EHR becomes a ubiquitous part of the practice.	Influences and manages the environment, does not "just adapt"
Allows EHR use to evolve; does not expect it to be ideal "out of the box."	Pragmatic, not idealistic
Recognizes that EHRs are the foundation for the future evolution of the practice (e.g., quality initiatives, electronic communication with the patient, health information exchange).	Future-oriented, not predominantly "present versus past" oriented
Creates a user environment for EHRs that enhances the relationship with the patient, the community and other healthcare providers.	Relationship-oriented, not just task-oriented
Adopts a philosophy that EHRs will improve connections to the community as well as process standardization to create greater internal integrity.	Embraces external connectivity and promotes internal integration

Table 3-2: Elements for Electronic Health Record (EHR) Success

many other things possible, such as improving efficiency, lowering costs, improving safety and so on.

Many practices are looking to improve efficiency because staffing costs are so high. By creating time lines and helping staff mark off important milestones, practice assimilation of the EHR becomes more concrete and clear. By using a phased-in, incremental approach to implementation, a connection to the past is maintained until it feels "safe" enough to use EHRs exclusively. Training and continual, consistent, concise communication create psychological safety in suddenly unfamiliar terrain. Customizing the new system to the practice's needs as well to staff's individual requirements allows the group to ensure cultural continuity.

There is no substitution for quality leadership during change or transition management. Groups that go forward without physician leadership quickly learn how essential that leadership is. It is essential that organizational leadership is synchronized with medical leadership. Demonstrating cohesiveness by developing clear, realistic goals for the project provides a solid foundation for the transition, decreases backsliding and ensures that the project will move forward positively. In preparation for EHRs, performing a readiness assessment allows the group to cooperate in identifying potential points of failure. A good offense is always more effective than a good defense.

In preparation for managing the transition, administrative and medical leadership must decide on clear, concise, cohesive messages. During times of transition, the practice constituency must be hearing a clear and continual message that is delivered consistently throughout the course of the project. Of course, the content that communication delivers varies based on individuals' roles and functions within the organization (i.e., the board of directors gets different communications than line staff).

When developing the message, the project team should be mindful of the following:

- **The focus is on continual improvement, not perfection.** Begin the message with a positive discussion of progress, specifically beginning with how far the practice has come. Next, the team can focus on the road ahead, namely where we want to be. Finally, lay out the short-, medium-, and long-term goals of the project and how we are going to get there. Include pertinent dates and schedules.

- **Identify where progress has been made and the role of each individual in contributing to that progress.** Begin the message with specific examples of progress, mentioning people and departments that have contributed to the progress. By the time the EHR system is live, all members of the staff should be mentioned—at least by department.

- **Change requires "unfreezing," which requires application of "heat."** Most organizations and people are adverse to conflict, making this concept one that is often hard to accept and incorporate. Groups need to focus on looking for specific symptoms or clues that adequate heat is being applied. This signal generally comes in the form of office "buzz"—what people are discussing "around the water cooler," so to speak. It can also come in the form of other symptoms that, if not addressed, can become destructive. Table 3-3 describes a framework for understanding when the "heat" has been turned up too high and how to cool it down by applying the right remedy. For example, using this model, if symptoms of confusion and conflict are observed, one might try to reaffirm and rearticulate the vision of the project. If there are symptoms of performance anxiety, adequate incentives for use of the system may have not been applied. If there is backsliding, perhaps adequate attention and time have not been applied to training and practice time. If there is frustration and anger, it is likely that additional training is needed to improve feelings of competence with the system. And, finally, if there are false starts, action plans must be addressed, reevaluated and adhered to.

Organizational Cultural Assessment Framework		
Observation	**Features of Culture**	**Interview**
What do the offices look like?	Ceremonies, rites, rituals	Tell me the organization's "creation story."
How are people dressed?	Stories, myths (e.g., stories told by managers about successes, failures)	How do new people "learn the ropes" here?
Where do people eat lunch?	Heroes, villains	What gets noticed (and rewarded)? Are some people on the "fast track"? If so, how did they get there? If a team accomplishes something great, what happens?
How would you characterize people in the halls?	Language, acronyms, metaphors	What are some organizational taboos—things people should never do?
What kinds of pictures, jokes and signs are on the walls?	Symbols, signs, logos	Describe the organization in three words.

Table 3-3: Organizational Cultural Assessment Framework

- **Change requires demonstrated commitment, not just compliance.** In *The Five Dysfunctions of a Team*,[2] Patrick Lencioni outlines a model that contains five dysfunctions which can be mistakenly interpreted as five distinct issues that can be addressed in isolation of the others. But in reality they form an interrelated model, making susceptibility to even one of them potentially lethal for the success of a team. The dysfunctions that deteriorate teamwork are
  1. Absence of trust;
  2. Fear of conflict;
  3. Lack of commitment;
  4. Avoidance of accountability; and
  5. Inattention to results.
  Developing an awareness of this model and how it can be applied within implementation teams is advisable, as it will lay a good foundation for optimal team functioning on future projects.

- **Feedback should be offered consistently and often.** In addition, it needs to be "packaged" in a way that it is perceived as a gift. Providing honest, kind and consistent feedback to staff is one of the most important responsibilities of leadership. A change of this magnitude often brings out the best and the worst behaviors—typically magnifying the worst. Actionable feedback compares "what is" to "what is expected" without judgment.

TRAINING

Most providers are intelligent, competent and self-directed individuals. They have also learned throughout their medical education and training to be demanding. Although intelligence, competence and self-direction are their greatest strengths, these traits can also be their greatest weaknesses because being in the role of student (again) is not easy for them. Experience tells us that providers easily become restless in training sessions and often have difficulty attending to one thing at a time.

In preparation for EHR adoption, leadership must communicate that system training is not optional and that all providers and staff are required to attend training. Furthermore, all employees are expected to practice the curriculum that has been taught. Prepare providers and staff to participate fully in classroom and on-the-floor training. Practice sessions should be monitored, and leadership needs to be prepared for those times when providers and staff are not compliant with training requirements. Providers do not easily submit to the role of student. Leadership must be prepared to use incentives, and possibly discipline, to encourage, cajole and/or demand that providers and staff attend training and practice sessions with an open mind and a willingness to learn.

DEVELOPING LEADERS

There is no substitute for leadership in a clinical transformation project. Preparing leaders ahead of the transformation improves the opportunity for success. Effective leaders are able to engage people to commit to company or practice goals. Too often leadership is defined mainly as an individual's ability to influence others. Although influence is certainly part of engaging others in a new process, it only tells part of the story. When it comes to leading during a time of enormous change, the transformational leadership style is the most effective.

Transformational leaders are described as charismatic leaders who take into consideration individual's characteristics and the needs of the constituency as a whole; also, these leaders can intellectually stimulate their constituents. Transformational leaders motivate others through values, vision and empowerment. Alternatively, *transactional leaders* tend to exchange rewards for efforts. However, long-term, second-order change does not seem to occur readily under transactional leadership. By definition, this type of leadership deals best with intermittent crises; it will not lead change that might protect the group from future crises. *Motivating leaders* selectively show their weakness, rely heavily on intuition, employ a "tough empathy" management style, and clearly differentiate themselves from the rest of their employees and staff.[3] A leader cannot compensate with a higher level of differentiation for a weak management style that avoids conflict and accepts mediocrity.

Furthermore, good leaders must be flexible and agile—able to adjust to a changing environment and new trends while maintaining a stable, predictable, and safe environment for employees and staff. People in leadership positions generally possess many skills. Among these may be intelligence, charisma, industry knowledge and specific talents. Knowing which skills to use and when to use them is what sets apart an effective, inspiring leader.

Prior to EHR implementation, learn how to identify leadership styles and select a medical leader for the project who demonstrates a transformational management style. This individual should have an awareness of various leadership styles and how to adopt new styles that are more useful during times of sweeping change. The provider leader may not be the most seasoned or obvious leader, however. Recognizing that different characteristics are needed based on the situation at hand improves the practice's opportunity for success. Look for leaders who are not afraid to show their own vulnerabilities; who are more interested in looking in the mirror when things go wrong and out the window when they are going right; who seem intuitively to understand the reasons for using EHRs; who demonstrate empathy and, at the same time, a tough, no nonsense demeanor; and who are less interested in being "friends" with everyone than in leading the group to the next level. Be prepared to address quickly any signs of vacillation that the EHR system is not the way to go or that the wrong vendor may have been chosen.

Too often administrators look to the most tech-savvy provider to lead the EHR project. However, tech savvy does not always mean that the individual is a strong, confident leader. Furthermore, any knowledge or skill gap in terms of IT can be bridged. Instead of giving extra weight to technology skills when considering who in the practice might be the best physician champion for the project, it is far better to err on the side of allowing strong leadership to trump IT proficiency. In the case of the physician who has very limited IT knowledge but who is a good candidate from the leadership perspective, plan on teaming him or her with someone else who is strong in IT skills. This partner can be a member of the technical team at the practice, an outsourced technology management services provider and/or a more tech savvy provider.

Are leaders born or made? Although this question cannot be answered here, what is clear is that effective leadership is not the result of a simple prescription or formula. Given the right mentoring environment, leadership skills can be developed and honed. In fact, in the words of Dwight D. Eisenhower, "The one quality that can be developed by studious reflection is the leadership of men."[4] In addition to the many characteristics described earlier, leaders must desire to lead and be willing to take on the responsibilities of leadership. Few people are willing to make the personal sacrifice of time and quality of life to be a good leader. Furthermore, the assumption that those who deliver results are the best leaders is also erroneous. Good leadership does not always equal good results, nor do good results automatically mean that good leadership was in place. The temptation is to look toward the most productive provider to lead important projects. However, good leadership may not be the reason behind his or her success.

Holding a leadership position either currently or in the past does not necessarily signify good leadership skills. Leadership, by definition, simply means there are followers. Reaching a leadership position may be more a function of exercising political acumen rather than actual leadership skills. In organizations where true leadership is lacking throughout, even the most lifeless person may rise to a leadership position—particularly in institutions that traditionally promote from within and are not expansive in their recruiting or worldly in their hiring practices.

Finally, good leaders are not always good coaches. Coaching assumes a set of technical skills and an in-depth knowledge that is highly specific to the task at hand (e.g., sports, life skills, parenting). Leadership is related more closely to the ability to inspire people to commit to a particular goal or set of objectives. Although good coaching is always needed, it is more important for big projects to inspire. Inspiration is the necessary ingredient that helps people stay focused and disciplined when the road to success is unclear or appears dangerous and treacherous. Effective leaders hire the staff they need to coach others (i.e., persons with effective management and technical expertise and in-depth knowledge in a particular subject area, such as IT). It is rare to find an effective leader who is also a good coach.

Integral to managing change and transition is the ability to inspire staff and partners to re-imagine the business of the organization in ways that allow the group to adapt to new ways of doing things, even when it feels uncomfortable or uncertain. Furthermore, organizations need this regular infusion of energy and vitality so they can embrace new ideas and concepts.

IT solutions are not nearly as pervasive in medical practices as they are in other businesses, and clearly, strong physician leadership can help with the transformation from paper-based to computerized systems. By far, the strongest influence on physicians is the word of their peers. Developing leaders within a practice may be the "tipping point" that guarantees successful EHR adoption. Leaders can focus on developing the following characteristics:

- Define a vision for the EHR and for the implementation project.
- Communicate the vision in multiple formats and using multiple vehicles (e.g., print, talks, graphics).
- Recognize leadership styles that are effective.
- Understand the difference between leadership and management.
- Learn and follow rules, within reason.
- Earn the trust of colleagues.
- Understand when to exercise power.
- Behave like a leader.
- Turn followers into leaders.
- Maintain personal balance.
- Strive to develop staff so that, eventually, the leader is no longer needed.[4]

"Vision is the currency of leadership."[4] Vision is what sets leadership apart from management. Managers are responsible for carrying out the leader's vision. This vision forms the organizational mission and motivates constituents. Communicating the vision clearly and concisely is the next essential step. This activity should be done formally and informally, in elevators and in the board room. It is important that everyone clearly understands the leader's vision for the organization. A shared vision is energizing and motivating.

Leadership styles can vary and, although there is no "right" way to lead, some styles are more effective than others. Recognized styles include autocratic or authoritarian, participative or democratic, and delegative or free reign. The autocratic/authoritarian style tends to expect compliance with orders because of the position of the leader. This style does not appreciate those who question the status quo and is most effective when stress is low and change is minimal or nonexistent. Participative or democratic leaders involve the stakeholders and constituency, gathering up the best ideas. Furthermore, the participative leader develops followers into leaders and focuses more on the organization than on personal gain. Finally, the delegative or free-reign style allows staff to make decisions independently. This style is best applied when staff have demonstrated good problem-solving skills. It can be utilized sparingly at first—giving staff the opportunity to develop key skills—and then used more liberally after staff have proven themselves.[4]

Effective leaders are able to distinguish leadership from management. Leaders do not run from risk; managers mitigate risk. Leaders minimize failures, focus on success, and inspire others with confidence. Because of their unyielding vision, leaders may appear to be set apart and living almost entirely in the future. Meanwhile, the manager is focused on the day to day.[4]

Rules, to a leader, provide a framework defining boundaries and identifying areas for innovation. Leaders use rules to their advantage, but they must take the time to learn official and unofficial rules. Although the leader may on occasion choose to break the rules, those rules are understood, known and respected.[4]

Trust is important, if not essential, to a well-functioning organization. To develop and engender trust, effective leaders make promises sparingly. However, when promises are made, they must be acted on in a timely fashion. Effective leaders have little to say and spend their time listening and soliciting information. No news is *not* good news in this instance. Effective leaders also clearly articulate and demonstrably live out their values. Where values are concerned, consistency is key.[4]

Power, like trust, is earned and granted from the constituency; it is not a function of position. Too often leaders simply assume power. They quickly realize, however, that power is meaningless without the endorsement of the people one is leading. A facilitative style that seeks to gain consensus allows for a more effective use of power.[4]

Leaders must always behave as leaders. They must live the values they expect and articulate because all eyes are on them. Everyone in the organization is watching the behavior of the leader. In one situation, for example, the CEO of the organization was seen "just standing by" while the chief operating officer tore into the chief financial officer in an inappropriate manner. The lack of response by the CEO and her seeming acceptance of that behavior was unsettling to staff and precipitated the resignation of at least one staff member. Constituents are looking for a leader to set the example and tone for the rest of the organization. Especially in the times of transition and change, such as when a new EHR system is implemented, the leader must be visible. Regular, consistent interaction puts staff at ease and mitigates the stress inevitably associated with major change.[4]

Leaders must not be threatened by budding leaders among their followers. A smart, competent, transformational leader develops those from the ranks who exhibit leadership qualities. Surrounding a leader with competent people who also have leadership qualities only improves the position of the leader and, ultimately, the organization.

Remember, the leader is more interested in the good of the organization than in personal gain. This quality confers the ultimate in confidence. Effective leaders develop and promote staff.[4]

Leaders are judged not only by their professional accomplishments, but also by their accomplishments outside their professional lives. Multiple failed relationships, an unhappy personal life, and the inappropriate use of the tobacco or alcohol, for example, undermine trust and confidence in one's leadership skills. Leaders must be prepared to demonstrate what they say. Again, all eyes are on the leader.[4]

RECOGNIZING LEADERSHIP QUALITIES

How can leadership potential be recognized and subsequently developed? Potential leaders have been in leadership positions in the past, either formally or informally, either in their work lives or in their personal lives (e.g., church, community). Potential leaders easily catch on to vision and are energized by it. A leader seeks out the thrill of a challenge. Most leaders are critical, but, at the same time, they offer alternative solutions; this is referred to as *constructive discontent*.

However, although innovation and original thinking are welcome, they are not necessarily the sign of a good leader. Leaders must be practical and consistently provide opportunities for the success for the constituency. Good leaders understand, appreciate, and demonstrate accountability. A good leader follows through and brings initiatives to completion. In addition to completing projects, a good leader does not necessarily need his/her idea to be the one that is adopted and developed. It is far more important and effective for the leader to plant the seed and provide a good environment for idea germination and growth. It is more effective because it leads to *second-level change*, which is sustaining and leads to the further growth and development of the organization. This approach requires patience because it is more time consuming and will be laden with trial and error. The leader must resist the temptation to jump in and solve the problem. The leader must learn to withhold counsel until just the right moment. This is a function of experience and self-discipline.

Leaders are mentally tough and can withstand criticism. They can separate being everyone's friend from earning the respect of peers. Finally, leaders command attention; when they speak, they are heard. Frequently, this is a phenomenon of listening often and speaking rarely. Good leaders have highly-developed listening skills; they ask a lot of questions and listen to the answers. They gather information and make decisions based on that information. There is a sense of openness and inclusiveness about an effective leader.

In the end, the physician champion will have many of the qualities of a leader. Physicians, as previously noted, are primarily motivated by their peers. The physician champion should not be confused with the project manager, however. The medical leader in collaboration with administrative leadership provides the vision, the guiding principles for the project, and, where necessary, uses power to enforce that vision. Conversely, the project manager implements that vision operationally. In fact, the project manager should regularly assign tasks to the physician champion.

In conclusion, physician champions and a group of individuals with leadership skills are essential to the success of EHR implementation. Physician champions can be developed when their leadership qualities are recognized and cultivated. Finally, sustainable second-order change is facilitated by a transformational leader—a leader who is charismatic, considers individual characteristics, considers the needs of the constituency and stimulates the constituency's intellect. A transformational leader does not accept the status quo. Instead, he/she is continually questioning the way things are and offering thoughtful, constructive solutions to problems that arise. Transformational leadership may require more patience, time, tolerance, and resources, but it is worth the wait.

LEARNING PATIENCE

Yes, this too shall pass. In the "thick" of EHR implementation, it is easy to lose perspective—"missing the forest for the trees" you are stumbling over every day. Prepare yourself for the difficult days to come by creating a support system that will help you maintain perspective:

- Select a champion who will be a good collaborator and communicator, who will help develop the vision, keeping in mind careful considerations of the practice culture and realistic expectations for the technology and how the message will be communicated.
- Talk to other administrators who are considered level-headed and who ultimately prevailed in EHR implementation. You will likely find that, although they might not have a "perfect" situation, they are continually making progress toward more efficient and effective processes.
- Identify potential saboteurs on management teams, be on the lookout for sabotage and remove saboteurs swiftly and decisively. Nothing torpedoes a good project more quickly than sabotage and leadership that tolerates it for too long.
- Develop a long-term vision and short-term tolerance for the disruptions caused by implementation. Try to act on project goals rather than the emotions stirred up by unhappy providers and staff. Consider using some outside consulting talent to help filter constructive feedback out of complaints.

CONCLUSION

EHR implementation is not for the faint of heart. It is hard work, has many "moving parts," and will impact every aspect of a medical practice. More than 50 percent of health IT projects fail. For the most part, such projects fail because practice leadership has been unrealistic about the impact of the change and the number of resources that must be committed to a project of this magnitude. Recognizing and embracing that EHR implementation is a change management project with an IT component is the first step toward ensuring project success. This recognition leads to greater awareness of organizational culture, intentional planning, and clear and consistent articulation of the vision and guiding principles of the project. In the end, these three areas can help to engage staff and improve the project's long-term chances for success.

REFERENCES

1.   Johnson S. *Who Moved My Cheese? An Amazing Way to Deal with Change in Your Work and in Your Life.* New York: Penguin Putnam; 2002.

2.   Lencioni P. *The Five Dysfunctions of a Team: A Leadership Fable.* San Francisco: Jossey-Bass; 2002.

3.   Goffee and Jones, 2000.

4.   Taylor RB. Leadership is a learned skill. *Family Practice Management* 2003; 10(9):43-48. http://www .aafp.org/fpm/2003/1000/p43.html. Accessed September 22, 2010.

CHAPTER 4

Proven, Field-Tested Strategies

INTRODUCTION

This chapter is devoted to various electronic health record (EHR) adoption strategies taken from experts, peers and early adopters. Given the transitional nature of EHR adoption, these tips and tricks are presented in the following order: (1) EHR readiness, (2) vendor selection, (3) implementation, and (4) optimization and enhancements.

EHR READINESS

Tip #1: Clearly document expectations for the project as well as goals and objectives. Although this tip seems basic, it is common for mistakes to happen later in the process because this step was overlooked. Some items for your list may include the following:

- Full integration with laboratories, diagnostic imaging and other test results.
- Works with the existing billing system.
- Proven for practice specialty.
- Structured documentation, integrations with transcription, point-and-click functionality, etc.
- 100 percent buy-in from all providers before beginning the vendor vetting process.
- Timing, budget, staffing and resources.

Tip #2: Use the self-assessment readiness guide in Appendix A to help establish expectations for the project as well as goals and objectives—and to avoid threats to the project's completion.

Tip #3: Become educated. Attend conferences, seminars and webinars, such as those provided by HIMSS, on the topic of EHR adoption. Visit a nearby practice that has recently undergone an EHR transformation and conduct online research to obtain information regarding how best to prepare for EHR adoption.

Tip #4: Start gathering information about how your practice captures, stores and retrieves data today. Examine how these processes might be impacted by an EHR and/ or how the system would need to address capturing, storing and retrieving this kind of data electronically. This task should be looked at from internal and external points of view. Consider these primary areas:

- Paper schedules
- Clinical notes
- Prescriptions, including narcotics
- Laboratories
- Referrals
- Information going to and from the hospital
- Ancillaries (electrocardiograms, radiology, etc.)
- Medication lists (current and discontinued)
- Messages and phone notes
- Reports
- Electronic data interchanges or clearinghouse
- Forms
  - Health Insurance Portability and Accountability Act of 1996
  - Intake
  - Clinical
  - New patients

Tip #5: Create a small workgroup to help formulate an adoption strategy and to help with project assessment. Eventually, this workgroup will be needed to help with vendor selection and project implementation, so organizing a good team early is helpful. Assign roles and responsibilities to the workgroup, such as defining key requirements for their departments (see details on project staffing in Appendix A).

Tip #6: Now is a good time to examine the practice's information technology (IT) infrastructure, such as the network, connectivity and workstations. An updated, modern network will be essential and should be looked at prior to launching any EHR initiative. This task will also help to establish a more accurate project budget.

Tip #7: Address staff anxiety and concerns. Although most staff members will be excited about getting a new EHR system, this change can be very threatening to some people. It is common for some staff members, especially those that work in medical records, to view EHRs as a threat to their job security. Although roles and responsibilities will be affected, rarely do EHR systems cause people to lose their jobs. The person who files paper today will likely be "repurposed" into an electronic scanning, archiving, and indexing role. Paper will still come into the practice and will need to be managed effectively.

Tip #8: Get physicians involved early. Specifically, any practice with more than one physician should identify a physician champion to take the lead as a project advocate and assist in overseeing decisions that have clear clinical implications. Larger practices might consider having a physician champion and a nonclinical executive sponsor or project manager who will help manage the project.

Tip #9: Do not prepare as if you are in a vacuum. Talk with other nearby practices that have been through this change to gather additional tips on this process and to learn what to expect.

Tip #10: Assign reading material and distribute articles about EHR selection to members of the workgroup.

Tip #11: As a rule, it is never wise to proceed to implementation until there is a basic level of acceptance toward the adoption of EHRs among all providers. It is common for some providers to be skeptical, or maybe even apprehensive, about EHRs. However, everyone should at least accept the concept—and real necessity—of automation before the practice starts this journey. Here are a few tips that might help you address providers who are reluctant to move forward:

- **The skeptical provider.** Suggest that this individual keep an open mind (although he/she is under no obligation) and at least consider looking at the technology so that he/she might play an active role in the process. Provide some education about how EHRs work and arrange for this provider to visit a practice with a successful EHR system in place. Ideally, it would be best to locate an EHR site where another provider was also previously skeptical.

- **The high-producing provider.** A highly productive provider can often be the most challenging person to win over to a new way of doing things. He/she may view the new system as a threat to income because the learning curve would slow down productivity, resulting in fewer patients seen. Although a productivity loss does occur in the beginning, generally, the pace should return to normal eventually. However, it is true that there are some providers with exceptionally high productivity levels that would be difficult to sustain with an EHR system. Under these circumstances, the provider must be convinced that income levels can remain the same despite seeing less patients if the EHR can help improve coding and reduce overhead costs. This is often a "hard sell" because these benefits are not immediate and can take months to realize. Several strategies can be implemented to reduce threats to high productivity, such as using a scribe, allowing dictation to flow into the EHR, using forms and then later scanning and abstracting the information. Avoiding future penalties, as tied to Medicare reimbursement reductions for not adopting EHRs, also can be used as a tool to help influence provider acceptance.

- **The near-retirement provider.** Physicians that are nearing retirement will often reject the concept of adopting an EHR because the cost does not justify the means this late in their careers. This objection is generally a nonissue for solo physicians in private practice with five or fewer years to retirement. However, even in late career, adopting an EHR can help the practice become more attractive when the retiring physician is ready to sell the practice. Physicians nearing retirement in a group practice can be more challenging to win over to EHRs because they often feel reluctant to share the cost of something they will not fully see the benefits from. Depending on the employment or operating agreement the practice has with the late-career physician, he/she may still be obligated to share the cost despite a negative opinion of the project. A compromise often reached in such situations is not to put the soon-retiring physician through a comprehensive implementation, knowing he/she will soon be leaving the practice. As a rule, the cost of an EHR system should be treated like any other operating expense—shared among all the physicians, regardless of their retirement status. If an exception occurs, it can result in everyone wanting similar "opt out" considerations on individual expenses they oppose. It is helpful to reinforce that everyone also shares in the benefits.

- **The unrealistic tech-savvy provider.** Yes, it is true. Even a tech-savvy provider can be reluctant to adopt an EHR. These individuals are searching for a system that is so technologically advanced that it simply does not exist. Alternatively, tech-savvy providers may have unrealistic expectations of the technology. This provider can also be intimidating to his or her peers and may be seen as over-ambitious. Visionaries throughout history often have been labeled as "fanatical" and have encountered challenges with getting their messages across to others. The tech-savvy provider must understand and accept that the goal is to help educate and lead those who are less familiar with technology than he/she is. These providers should be encouraged not to communicate with a "techie" vocabulary (e.g., lots of acronyms) to those who are new to EHRs.

- **The unengaged provider.** Although some physicians accept the concept of EHRs, they will not participate in the process. Alternatively, they will take the classic passive position of just going along with whatever the group wants to do. These same providers will often wait until after decisions have been made to voice their opinions. A role can be created for this type of provider to ensure participation in the process. Some practices require big decisions, such as adopting an EHR system, to come to a vote. This protocol forces each physician to make a yes or no decision. It is also often helpful to provide lots of information to physicians throughout the process to avoid being later accused of not informing them.

- **The Lone Ranger provider.** Although rare, some practices have encountered a situation where a single provider will grow impatient with a group's lack of responsiveness to adopting an EHR and will go off and purchase something on his/her own. This tactic can be extremely disruptive to the process and it can create several conflicts. Depending on the group's structure and governance policies, this behavior should not be tolerated or accepted as a constructive way to get the group to adopt an EHR. It can also be precarious, allowing the provider to keep his/her EHR temporarily until the group makes a formal decision. Taking away a physician's personal EHR system is never pleasant.

VENDOR SELECTION

Chapter 6 is devoted to vendor vetting and selection. Following are additional tips for a successful vendor transaction.

Tip #1: Prescreen vendors with some basic questions before inviting them into the formal screening process. This step will save time and money by allowing you to avoid situations where vendors clearly do not meet expectations.

Tip #2: Have vendors send information about their companies and products in advance to distribute to the workgroup so everyone will be familiar with the companies before their representatives arrive.

Tip #3: Avoid offers of expensive dinners, gifts or paid trips to avoid undue influence in the decision-making process.

Tip #4: Take time to set expectations with vendors in advance. If time permits, have them come to the practice to review your operations and workflow prior to the demonstration. This time-saving tip will give vendors the opportunity to specifically address your needs and customize their demonstration to the goals and objectives of the practice.

Tip #5: Get a list of references early and begin to seek information. Most people wait until the end of the selection process to obtain references. Start talking to others that use the same system as soon as possible to find out quickly if the vendor is living up to expectations with its customers.

Tip #6: Use a demonstration script. A sample demonstration script is included in Appendix A.

Tip #7: Consider having the vendor do the demonstration in the examination room with an actual patient. The vendor would serve as scribe while the physician is examining the patient. (Prior patient approval is recommended.)

Tip #8: Go off site to hold product demonstrations so that they are not disruptive to the practice. Off-site review also allows for greater focus during product evaluation. Start late afternoon and end around 7:00 PM. Try to schedule two or three vendors per session.

Tip #9: Use scorecards and evaluation tools. See Appendix A on tools for several examples.

Tip #10: Leave time for hands-on interaction and ask the vendor to conduct some mock simulations using actual scenarios played out by staff members.

Tip #11: Have each member of the workgroup come prepared with a list of questions. Send these questions to the vendor in advance so they can come prepared to answer and demonstrate the software accordingly.

Tip #12: Count clicks. Pay close attention to how many clicks and screens it takes for the system to perform a certain function. Too many clicks can slow down a provider.

Tip #13: Examine the ability of providers to customize the system on the fly. This flexibility will be critical to successful adoption. The system should be easily customizable to meet the needs of the provider.

Tip #14: Look for navigation shortcuts and workflow options. A good system should allow the user to get around the application easily and into different areas of the EHR without going through a lot of steps. A well-designed system will often resemble an Internet browser that allows users to move around within the application yet maintain the exact same navigation tools throughout the record.

Tip #15: Look for a system that provides point-of-care feedback, such as decision support tools. Even simple things like the hourglass symbol to indicate when the system is "thinking" or locating information is helpful to the end user. Error messages, alerts, and required fields are also examples of system feedback that will be helpful to the end user.

Tip #16: Does the system have built-in learning tools and online help resources? Can the vendor access the system remotely to observe/fix the issues you encounter? Can they provide remote training by taking over system controls in real time to demonstrate how to use key features?

Tip #17: Look for features that allow data from past visits to be reused and/or pulled forward. This is a significant time saver for physicians who care for patients with chronic conditions.

Tip #18: Clearly understand what is included in the system being considered and demonstrated. Many vendors will demonstrate features that are add-ons purchased separately. Make it clear to vendors that they are not to demonstrate any add-on features without first identifying them as being available at an extra cost.

Tip #19: Make sure to inspect the vendors' standard reports and compare these reports to your practice's current requirements and expectations. Most often, custom reports are done at an extra expense and may be difficult to modify once the system is configured. Also, see if the vendor has a "dashboard" report to display critical performance standards and vital signs about utilization of the system.

Tip #20: Avoid creative financing offers, such as deferred payments, unless you are fully prepared to pay off the system despite any unforeseen circumstances. Failure to pay could result in the lender modifying terms and interest rates or calling the balance of the loan to be paid in full.

Tip #21: Take time to review and negotiate your vendor contract and terms. Chapter 8 is devoted to vendor negotiations. So the tip here is to read Chapter 8 twice to make sure vendor contracting and negotiating strategies are clearly understood. Here are some additional vendor negotiating tips:

- Compare quotes from vendors. Comparing vendor pricing can be challenging because you will not always have apples-to-apples comparisons. For example, Vendor A may include third-party software, such as a Microsoft-based operating system, in their final price. Vendor B does not include this operating system in their quote even though it is required. This omission gives the illusion that Vendor B is less expensive, when, in fact, their services will cost much more after cost of the third-party software is added into their totals.
- Pay close attention to recurring fees and vendor add-on services.
- Ask the vendor if they will give you a guarantee not to exceed budget.
- Get everything in writing and keep all the documentation and e-mails related to system/vendor promises organized and readily accessible. The salesperson making the promises may leave the company. This documentation will be helpful to support your argument, if necessary.
- Require the vendor to itemize all expenses, including implementation. Some vendors will show a lump sum budget of hours for training and implementation. Have the vendor provide the details on how these hours will be used. The invoices they send should include a similar level of detail.
- Require the vendor to provide a sample project plan and implementation schedule prior to contracting to verify that it matches the project budget and staff expectations.
- Vendors generally give discounts that range from 15 to 40 percent off, so do not be afraid to ask—especially when purchasing multiple products from the same vendor, such as a combination PM/EHR system.
- Make sure you have a good warranty. (Chapter 8 addresses warranties more specifically.)

- Never pay in full for any service in advance. Payment terms should always be tied to project objectives and accomplishments. This condition is true for additional services as well, including interfacing, data conversions, and custom reports. Typically it is fair to agree to pay a percentage up front, but the bulk of the payment should be due on successful completion of the deliverable. Most vendors request 50 percent at signing and 50 percent on completion. (Chapter 8 presents and recommends a more granular payment schedule that places most of the compensation on the back end, after completion and implementation of the bulk of the work.)
- Know and understand the type of software license you are purchasing. Your vendor may propose any of the following options:
  - **Term license.** Allows use of the software for a limited period of time. Under this type of license, you do not own the software; you have only purchased the right to use it while under contract with the vendor.
  - **Purchase license.** Under this kind of arrangement, you fully own the license and do not have any obligation to be under contract.
  - **Perpetual license.** A license of this kind is based on the number of people that can use the system at any given time. A perpetual license is good for practices with a large number of employees or part-time providers.
  - **Software as a service (SaaS).** This licensing option allows the client to obtain a subscription to the software. Generally, this option requires no up-front capital cost.

Tip #22: The Office of the National Coordinator for Health Information Technology (ONC) published regulations detailing the process for EHR vendors to obtain a Certified System designation. Vendors will need to meet these standards to qualify for Certified EHR status. Physicians must select from among these approved systems if they wish to participate in the EHR financial incentive program through the American Recovery and Reinvestment Act of 2009 (ARRA). To qualify for stimulus incentives, the practice must select a system that conforms to the standards set by ONC. Since not all standards are currently known, it is essential to have your vendor provide an EHR certification warranty to ensure your practice's eligibility for stimulus funds.

Following is a sample EHR certification warranty that you may want to consider adding to your vendor contract:

> All versions of the electronic health record (EHR) necessary to satisfy all requirements to be considered a Certified EHR (as defined below) for use by Client to receive all of the Medicare or Medicaid incentives available under the Health Information Technology for Economic and Clinical Health Act (HITECH) beginning on October 1, 2010, and will not be subject to any reduction in reimbursement as a result of a failure to meet "certified EHR requirements" necessary to qualify for Meaningful Use.

> As used herein, the terms "Certified EHR," "Meaningful Use," and "meaningful user" each have the respective meanings assigned to such terms in HITECH (and any subsequent amendments thereto, including stages 1 to 5) and in the regulations to be determined from time to time pursuant

to HITECH, including whichever are then the most recent versions of HITECH and such regulations that become required.

Vendor agrees to provide all implementation, training, data conversion, and other services that may be necessary or appropriate to reasonably assist Client in implementing each of the Certified EHR versions that Client may, in its discretion, elect to implement in becoming a meaningful user.

All modules necessary to comply as a Certified EHR—such as eRx, patient portals, continuity-of-care records, and health information exchange integration—will be provided at no additional charge to the Client.

IMPLEMENTATION

The implementation phase often requires some skillful interpersonal tactics. Please review the following tips:

Tip #1: Create some excitement and model how to have fun with the project. Perhaps get some t-shirts made for the EHR crew doing the implementation work. Regularly post countdown signs around the office to promote the go-live date as the big event.

Tip #2: Provide food and treats for staff when working after regular office hours. Allow for some rest or compensation time to make up the difference. Burnout can happen easily during the implementation stage. Allowing time for staff to take a break from the process will help your practice avoid this pitfall.

Tip #3: Post signs in the examination rooms and waiting room asking patients for their understanding and patience as the office undergoes the transition to EHRs. The sign should be similar to the apologetic "pardon our dust" signs often seen during facility construction and remodeling projects.

Tip #4: Name your project or system. I know this sounds inconsequential, but calling it "an IT project" or "EHR implementation" sounds boring and uninteresting. "The quality-improvement project" and "the modernization project" are examples that will help staff members see the project as being important.

Tip #5: Similar to the vendor-selection team, create an implementation team that consists of team members with different skills and perspectives.

Tip #6: Conduct a pre-implementation survey to gather information about staff concerns, expectations and goals or objectives.

Tip #7: When possible, dedicate an area of the office as a workroom/training room. Add a whiteboard, flip charts, projector and workstations to the training room.

Tip #8: Add some variety to the training methodology. Not everyone learns the same way. For example, provide reading materials, online tools, training guides, peer-to-peer sessions, and workshops. Your vendor should have tools to help you with this part of the project.

Tip #9: Create live training simulations and conduct rehearsals using staff members as mock patients to help verify skills and to test processes.

Tip #10: Designate "super users" early. These are advanced users who receive additional training and who will often learn special skills, such as system modification.

Tip #11: Avoid the temptation to start customizing the system before learning the basics. Although some customization will be needed, it is best to understand the basics thoroughly so that customization does not duplicate built-in features. In other words, customization is not a good way to make up for a lack of training. Early customization is almost always a sign of inadequate training—or an incomplete system.

Tip #12: Develop realistic project goals and objectives and create ways to measure progress toward these goals.

Tip #13: Set a realistic time line. Then, add several additional months to accommodate unexpected delays. Setting unrealistic time lines and goals, even when done inadvertently, will create feelings of failure when these goals are not achieved.

Tip #14: Forecast and budget resources based on the needs of the project. You do not want to find yourself going into the final week of training only to have your lead trainer going on a two-week vacation. Also, budget time for unexpected delays and delays that are completely outside of your control. For example, upgrading the Internet connection is usually done by the telephone company, which does not always work on your schedule. Creating a flexible resource schedule will help everyone avoid frustration and unnecessary feelings of failure. Other budget items to consider when resource planning:

- Meetings
- Vendors and technical experts coming into the office
- Time to go off-site to visit other practices
- Vacations, sick days, and inclement weather
- Other unexpected delays

Tip #15: Involve leadership and make them visible and available throughout the EHR adoption process. Even in practices with one physician, it is important that leaders remain involved and supportive as the practice makes the transformation.

Tip #16: Develop implementation plans with input from the vendor as well as practices that have been through the process already.

Tip #17: Consider hiring a consultant that specializes in EHR implementation. Some vendors can recommend consultants who are certified on their software.

Tip #18: Devote a project manager to oversee the entire process. The project manager should have the following fundamental skills:

- Good problem-solving skills
- Healthcare operations and workflow knowledge, especially clinical workflow
- Effective organizational skills
- Good communication skills
- Positive attitude
- Ability to take "push back" from others without taking it personally
- Ability to delegate and multitask
- Good leadership skills
- Respected by peers

Tip #19: Use tools, such as status reports, project budgets, implementation plans, and written policies and procedures, to communicate project status to staff.

Tip #20: Create a "design, build, and validation" (DBV) process. This is an industry-wide implementation model and is considered a "best practice" for EHR adoption. The process is simple and creates some essential checks and balances. In addition, undergoing this process helps reduce the possibility of going live with an untested or incomplete system. Basically, it works like this:

- **Design.** A team of subject matter experts familiar with the requirements of a certain functionality requirement will design the required workflow without any concern of how the system will respond to the requested requirements. This team is designing workflow around best practices and the ability to optimize productivity for the department or specific requirement.
- **Build.** A software expert will build and design the system based on input from the design team. Usually, this is done with the help of the vendor.
- **Validation.** After the build is complete, the design team reviews and validates the work by running a mock exercise or simulated scenario to test the new system. Minor tweaks are usually required.

Tip #21: Conduct ongoing testing, validation and optimization.

Tip #22: Watch out for "scope creep." Scope creep occurs when the scope or vision of a project expands beyond its budget and other planned resources. Scope creep can cause project failure by expanding the project beyond the budget or expected required resources. Creating an approval process for any services that lie outside the scope of the project will help prevent scope creep. Have no fear when holding the vendor accountable for causing scope creep.

Tip #23: Use vendor contract payment terms to help ensure the vendor meets performance objectives.

Tip #24: Interfacing applications can be a challenge, but when done correctly, it can be a tremendous enhancement to any EHR. Common interface applications include outbound laboratory orders, inbound laboratory results, dictation/transcription, radiology images and reports, hospital admissions and discharge summaries, and diagnostic results (electrogardiogram, pulse oximetry).

OPTIMIZATION AND ENHANCEMENTS

Optimizing an EHR is taking it to the next level of efficiency and productivity within your practice. Optimization begins when users start experimenting and having fun with the new system. Your vendor is your best source for seeking out enhancement tips specific to your system. Some of the tips listed in this section are software-dependent and may not be possible within the software you have chosen.

Tip #1: Create "exploding" diagnosis codes. Many EHR systems allow you to design a standard treatment plan tied to a specific diagnosis code. Then, when the diagnosis code is entered in the system, the entire treatment plan—complete with orders, documentation, and follow-up instructions—automatically populates the physician notes section of the EHR form. This enhancement is usually best applied to diagnoses for which treatment plans do not have a lot of variation (e.g., insect bites).

Tip #2: Use point-of-care charge-capturing to code and bill for services. This feature allows the provider to enter charges as they see each patient, eliminating manual charge entry and paper "super bills." Most systems provide point-of-care feedback based on the level of code contrasted against the documentation. Although this is a helpful feature, providers should always be aware that they are ultimately responsible for accurate coding, especially for Medicare patients.

Tip #3: Add a patient portal to the system. A patient portal allows patients to interact with the EHR remotely by giving them access to information defined by the practice. The portal can allow patients to request appointments, request prescription refills, print off their own medical records, and pay bills online.

Tip #4: Consider adding a patient kiosk to the waiting room. A kiosk allows for self-check-in, much like those that are available at airports. The kiosk can also take information from patients to help minimize routine questions during examinations. In addition, patients can make their copayments in advance, while they are waiting to be seen by a provider.

Tip #5: Add smart devices, such as handheld charge-capturing, smartphone integration, voice recognition, speech microphone, iPad, etc.

Tip #6: Build a network that allows for safe and secure remote access to protect against intrusions and security breaches. Protecting patient data should be a top priority with all EHRs.

Tip #7: Customize templates and create workflow tools, such as phone notes, triage scripts and patient education materials.

Tip #8: Participate in incentive programs, such as the Physician Quality Reporting Initiative and eRx. However, eRx incentives cannot be combined with ARRA's EHR stimulus incentives. Consider contacting your malpractice insurance carrier who can often provide discount incentives for adopting EHRs. Vendors may also consider offering "good customer" discounts to encourage staff to obtain certified training.

Tip #9: Master the reporting features in your EHR and start using the data to make business decisions and begin optimizing practice profitability. Having an EHR gives you the opportunity to look at information differently. For example, you can find out how many patients are overdue for routine health maintenance examinations and provide patient reminders. You can also measure your quality indicators as evidence of cost reductions for payers, which can be helpful during contract negotiations.

CONCLUSION

Successful EHR implementation is the result of sound strategy and good luck. Because EHRs are continually evolving, the journey to the "perfect" EHR system is never complete. New technologies and new regulations influence how these systems operate and how we are required to use them. Medical practices are faced with many new challenges—and also new opportunities. Implementing an EHR is a great opportunity to reinvigorate a practice and to spur it on toward new levels of success.

Our final tip, however, for this chapter is to have *fun*—and do not get discouraged. You are not alone and no method or system is perfect. Whatever works best for your practice and encourages maximal adoption and optimization will define your measure of success.

CHAPTER 5

EHR Compliance and Incentives

INTRODUCTION

Compliance and incentive issues relating to electronic health records (EHRs) is an extremely difficult subject to cover in the context of a book, as regulations and policies continue to evolve and undergo change. Even more challenging, this book is being written in the midst of sweeping new healthcare regulations, policies and mandates, combined with healthcare reform—the largest single policy change in our nation's history. The information here, accessed in December 2010, is from the official EHR Incentive Program website (www.cms.gov/EHRIncentivePrograms/), published by the Centers for Medicare & Medicaid Services (CMS). This website is specifically designed to provide official EHR incentive information and updates as they become available.

The website features resources, tools and guides to help practices stay on top of the Health Information Technology for Economic and Clinical Health (HITECH) Act incentives and requirements for participation. These resources are from official government sources, enabling users who frequently revisit the site to obtain updates during their transformation to EHR adoption.

WHERE WE ARE TODAY

The nation's healthcare system is undergoing transformation at every level in an effort to improve quality, safety and efficiency of care. This transformation ranges from massive undertakings, such as upgrading the entire ICD-10 coding system to information exchanges of EHR technology. To help facilitate this vision, the HITECH Act established programs under Medicare and Medicaid to provide incentive payments for the "meaningful use" of certified EHR technology. The Medicare and Medicaid EHR Incentive Programs will provide incentive payments to eligible professionals and eligible hospitals as they adopt, implement, upgrade or demonstrate meaningful use of certified EHR technology. The incentive programs, which begin in 2011, are designed to support providers in this period of health IT transition and instill the use of EHRs in meaningful ways to achieve nationwide improvement in the quality, safety and efficiency of patient healthcare.

According to the CMS Medicare and Medicaid EHR Incentive Programs website, CMS and the Office of National Coordinator for Healthcare Information Technology (ONC) underwent an extensive process for establishing the EHR Incentive Programs through formal rule making. The EHR Incentive Programs (and the definition of meaningful use) was published in early 2010; CMS accepted public comments for a 60-day period ending March 15, 2010. More than 2,000 comments were received.[1] Organizations such as HIMSS, the American Medical Association and major health systems provided input and served on committees to develop the initial requirements. On July 28, 2010, CMS published the final rule, which provides many of the parameters and requirements for the Medicare & Medicaid EHR Incentive Program. A copy of the final rule and related documents are accessible on the official EHR Incentive Programs website.[1]

GETTING STARTED

As noted, policies are subject to change, or new policies are apt to be added. For certain, ONC will publish five years of additional meaningful use guidance and requirements. As of October 2010, the official EHR incentive website offered the following recommendations for getting started with participating in the EHR Incentive Programs under the HITECH Act:[1]

The Medicare and Medicaid EHR Incentive Programs provide a financial reward for the meaningful use of qualified, certified EHRs to achieve health and efficiency goals. By implementing a certified EHR system, providers will reap benefits beyond financial incentives—such as reduction in errors, availability of records and data, reminders and alerts, clinical decision support, and e-Prescribing/refill automation.[1]

Key words in the above statement from CMS include the use of a "Certified EHR" in a "meaningful way," specifically, to achieve certain health and efficiency goals. This underscores the necessity to ensure your vendor complies with these standards and the system is implemented in a way to support the objectives. Merely buying an EHR will not qualify a provider for incentive payments.

INCENTIVE PROGRAM OVERVIEW

Incentive programs vary significantly between Medicare and Medicaid. Moreover, some policies prohibit participating in more than one program. For example, an eligible provider cannot participate concurrently in e-Prescribing incentives and EHR stimulus incentives. As of today, the Stark law is still relaxed for hospitals that seek to financially subsidize the purchase of an EHR for their non-employed medical staff. Following is a summary of incentive programs for providers under the Original Medicare (fee-for-service), Medicare Advantage, and Medicaid programs:

Medicare will provide incentive payments to eligible professionals (EPs) and eligible hospitals that demonstrate meaningful use of certified EHR technology. Requirements for becoming an EP are discussed in more detail later in this chapter. Starting in 2011, eligible professionals that demonstrate meaningful use using a certified EHR can receive up to $44,000 over five years under the Medicare incentive program. There are additional incentives for eligible professionals who provide services to the underserved and that have at least 30 percent of patients being seen under **Medicaid**. Medicaid EHR incentive programs are voluntarily offered by individual states and territories and may begin in 2011. Eligible professionals can receive up to $63,750 over the six years that they choose to participate in the program. Eligible professionals that participate in **Medicare Advantage** are also qualified to participate in the EHR incentive program. In addition, CMS will provide incentive payments for certain Medicare Advantage Organizations (MAOs) whose affiliated eligible professionals demonstrate meaningful use, utilizing certified EHR technology.

WHAT YOU NEED TO PARTICIPATE IN THE EHR INCENTIVE PROGRAMS

As noted above, buying just any EHR and using an EHR does not guarantee qualification. There are two critical requirements.
1.   Must use a certified EHR as determined and approved by ONC.
2.   Must use the EHR in a meaningful way as determined by CMS.

Specifically each eligible provider must comply with the following:

Certified EHR Technology

In order to qualify for an EHR incentive payment, all eligible professionals and hospitals need to have implemented a certified EHR technology. The standards for certified EHR technology, now available, establish the required capabilities that certified EHR technology will need to include to support the achievement of meaningful use. For vendors to become certified, they must meet requirements defined by ONC. A list of these qualified vendors can be found on the ONC website (http://healthit.hhs.gov).[1]

As discussed previously, vendors should also provide a stimulus guarantee/warranty. To learn more about certified EHR technology, see the CMS website.[1]

NOTE: You do not need to have your certified EHR in place in order to register for the EHR incentive programs. However, you must have adopted, implemented, upgraded, or meaningfully use certified EHR technology before you will receive an EHR incentive payment from either Medicare or your State Medicaid Agency. For more information on the years to participate in the program and possible incentive payments, go to the official EHR Incentive Programs website and click on the link titled "Medicare Eligible Professional." The eligible professional rules vary under Medicare and Medicaid. For example, under Medicaid, mid-level providers such as nurse practitioners are eligible for incentives, but they are not under Medicare. This is covered in more detail later in this chapter.

HOW TO ENROLL

To participate, eligible hospitals and eligible professionals must have a National Provider Identifier (NPI). If you are an eligible professional but do not have an NPI and/or a National Plan and Provider Enumeration System (NPPES) web user account, NPI-NPPES information is available at www.cms.gov/NationalProvIdentStand. At this site, you can apply for an NPI and/or create a NPPES user account.

All eligible hospitals and Medicare eligible professionals must also be enrolled in the CMS Provider Enrollment, Chain and Ownership System (PECOS) to participate in the EHR incentive program. Most will also need an active user account in the NPPES.

CMS will use these systems' records to register providers for the program and verify enrollment information prior to making incentive program payments. CMS will not come out to your office to verify the installation, but they can audit, which may result in an on-site inspection and/or they may request documentation of participation such as proof of purchase. For more information about PECOS enrollment, go to "Medicare Provider & Supplier Enrollment" at http://www.cms.gov/MedicareProviderSupEnroll/. In addition, the PECOS enrollment form is available at the CMS Medicare and Medicaid EHR Incentive Programs website.[1]

NOTE: Medicaid eligible professionals who are only participating in the Medicaid EHR incentive program are not required to enroll in PECOS.[1]

WHAT YOU CAN DO NOW

Other programs related to the EHR incentive programs provide technical assistance and best practices in EHR adoption and meeting meaningful use. To learn more about Regional Extension Centers, Beacon Communities, State Health Information Exchange Cooperative Agreement partners, and what is happening to further the adoption of health IT, visit ONC's website (http://healthit.hhs.gov).

Eligibility

The following guidelines are required for meeting Meaningful Use eligibility:[1]

In order to participate in the Medicare and Medicaid EHR incentive programs, health professionals and hospitals must meet the eligibility criteria defined by law. Eligibility groups are listed below.

Eligibility for Individual Providers – Eligible Professionals (EPs)

The incentives for eligible professionals are based on individual providers. Therefore, if you are part of a practice, each eligible professional may qualify for an incentive payment provided they successfully demonstrate meaningful use. Each EP is only eligible for one incentive payment each year, regardless of the number of practices or locations at which they provide services.

Medicare: A Medicare EP is defined as a doctor of medicine or osteopathy, doctor of dental surgery or dental medicine, doctor of podiatry, doctor of optometry or a chiropractor who is not hospital-based.

NOTE: A Medicare EP is considered hospital-based if 90% or more of the EP's services are performed in a hospital inpatient or emergency room setting.

Medicaid: A Medicaid EP is defined as a physician, nurse practitioner, certified nurse-midwife, dentist, or physician assistant who furnishes services in a Federally Qualified Health Center or Rural Health Clinic that is led by a physician assistant. To qualify for an EHR incentive payment, a Medicaid EP must not be hospital-based and must meet one of the following criteria:

- Have a minimum 30% Medicaid patient volume*
- Have a minimum 20% Medicaid patient volume, and is a pediatrician*
- Practice predominantly in a Federally Qualified Health Center or Rural Health Center and have a minimum 30% patient volume attributable to needy individuals

NOTE: A Medicaid EP is considered hospital-based if 90% or more of the EP's services are performed in a hospital inpatient or emergency room setting.

A provider who is employed by the hospital, but performs his or her services in an ambulatory setting is NOT considered hospital based.

EPs Eligible for Both Programs

If you are an EP that is eligible for both the Medicare and the Medicaid incentive program, you can only participate in one program, not both. You will need to select the program you want to participate in when you register.

Here are the general guidelines explaining the differences:

Medicare EHR Incentive Program	Medicaid EHR Incentive Program
Can participate as soon as the federal program launches January 1, 2011	Can participate once my state offers the program (check with your state for expected launch date)
Can receive up to $44,000 in incentives, and up to $48,400 if practicing in a Health Provider Shortage Area	Can receive up to $63,750 in incentives
Required to demonstrate meaningful use of certified EHR technology for 90 days in first year of the program and then for one year to qualify for payment	Can qualify for payment for adopting, implementing, upgrading or demonstrating meaningful use of certified EHR technology in first participation year. Required to demonstrate meaningful use in each subsequent year to qualify for payment.
Must participate by the second year to receive the maximum incentive payment	Must participate by 2016 to receive the maximum incentive payment

NOTE: Before 2015, an eligible professional may switch between the Medicare and Medicaid incentive programs one time after the first incentive payment is initiated.[1]

Medicare Advantage Organization Eligible Professionals: The Medicare Advantage EHR incentive program is structured differently than the Medicare EHR incentive program for Medicare Fee-for-Service providers. The official CMS EHR Incentive Programs website provides more details for qualifying under Medicare Advantage.

---

* Children's Health Insurance Program (CHIP) patients do not count toward the Medicaid patient volume criteria.

CERTIFICATION

The term "certification" surfaces frequently when considering required qualifications for EHR adoption and eligibility for receiving stimulus incentives. Just as guidelines have been established for how to use the EHR, there is an extensive set of guidelines for determining what qualifies as a "certified" EHR. The official EHR incentive website describes certification as the following:

Providers and patients must be confident that the electronic health information technology (IT) products and systems they use are secure, can maintain data confidentially, can work with other systems to share information, and can perform a set of well-defined functions. To this end, standards, implementation specifications, and certification criteria for health IT are being established by ONC.[1]

ONC has also created a list of vendor requirements, and it engaged public comment through formal rule making as a way to finalize these standards and criteria. This process took more than a year and in early 2010, ONC published an interim final rule on the standards and certification criteria and accepted public comments. ONC released its final rule on July 13, 2010, which established the required capabilities, related standards and implementation specifications that certified EHR technology will need to include, at a minimum, support the achievement of meaningful use Stage 1. A list of these requirements is published on ONC's website.

The goal of ONC is to assure that certified EHR technology for the incentive programs will be capable of performing the required procedures for meaningful use Stage 1 in order to qualify for incentive payments. This also forces all vendors to conform to uniform standards, clearing the way for integration and exchange of information, similar to the way our financial systems work. Vendors must prove their system can comply with these standards by undergoing an inspection and audit by an approved ONC-certifying agency, such as CCHIT.

Note: ONC has several certifying agencies; these approved agencies are listed on ONC's website.

As of the writing of this chapter, more than 50 vendors have been certified and more are being added to the list each month. It is anticipated that recertification will be required each year as the meaningful use guidelines evolve and become more comprehensive. Therefore, vendors must not only guarantee compliance during the first year, but also for future years. This can be a difficult dilemma for vendors since these future requirements are not yet known.

For more information on vendor certification requirements and certification standards, see ONC's website (http://healthit.hhs.gov).

HOW CERTIFICATION IS RELATED TO THE EHR INCENTIVE PROGRAMS

As noted previously, the EHR Incentive Programs require the use of both certified EHR technology and the demonstration of meaningful use. Accordingly, system functionality standards have been established. Existing EHR technology requires certification by an ONC-Authorized Testing and Certification Body (ONC-ATCB) to meet these new criteria in order to qualify for the incentive payments. It is recommended that your vendor provide you with a warranty to guarantee their software/products comply with these standards. Using an EHR that is not certified will disqualify you from participating in the incentive program.

Note: You do not have to have your certified EHR in place in order to register for the EHR incentive programs. Enrollment is now open and is available to anyone who meets the requirements. Nevertheless, you must have adopted, implemented, upgraded or meaningfully use certified EHR technology before you will receive a payment from either Medicare or Medicaid.

MEANINGFUL USE

The most critical component to qualifying for EHR incentives is the need to meet the meaningful use requirements. Simply put, the EHR must be used in a way that produces meaningful outcomes and results geared at lowering cost and improving patient care. Currently, the official EHR incentive website defines meaningful use as follows:

The Medicare and Medicaid EHR incentive programs provide a financial reward for the meaningful use of qualified, certified EHRs to achieve health and efficiency goals. By implementing and meaningfully using an EHR system, providers will reap benefits beyond financial incentives—like reduction in errors, availability of records and data, reminders and alerts, clinical decision support and e-Prescribing/refill automation.

To qualify for incentive payments, meaningful use requirements must be met in the following ways:

- **Medicare EHR Incentive Program** – Eligible professionals and hospitals must successfully demonstrate meaningful use of certified EHR technology every year they participate in the program.
- **Medicaid EHR Incentive Program** – Eligible professionals and hospitals may qualify for incentive payments for the adoption, implementation, upgrade or the demonstration of meaningful use in their first year of participation. They must successfully demonstrate meaningful use for the remaining years they participate in the program.[1]

DEFINITION OF MEANINGFUL USE REQUIREMENTS

As noted above, the meaningful use requirements were released on July 13, 2010. The final rule outlines all the specifics of Stage 1 meaningful use and clinical quality measure reporting to receive the incentive payments in 2011 and 2012.

The American Recovery and Reinvestment Act of 2009 specifies three main components of Meaningful Use:

- The use of a certified EHR in a meaningful manner (e.g., e-Prescribing);
- The use of certified EHR technology for electronic exchange of health information to improve quality of healthcare; and
- The use of certified EHR technology to submit clinical quality and other measures.

The definition of meaningful use harmonizes criteria across CMS programs as much as possible and coordinates with existing CMS quality initiatives. It also closely links to the certification standards criteria in development by ONC and provides a platform for a staged implementation over time.[1]

Specifics of Stage 1 Meaningful Use

Meaningful use for eligible professionals includes 25 meaningful use objectives. Of the 25 objectives, there are 20 core objectives that must be completed to qualify for an incentive payment; 15 are mandatory core objectives that are required, and the remaining five objectives may be chosen from the list of 10 menu set objectives.

To help with the adoption and transition to these new standards, the criteria for meaningful use will be staged in three steps over the course of the next five years. Stage 1 sets the baseline for electronic data capture and information sharing. Stage 2 is expected to be released in 2013, and Stage 3 will be released by 2015. It is also predicted that CMS will continue to expand on this baseline and it will be developed through future rule making. More information about meaningful use and the adoption stages can be found at the CMS website.[1]

At the end of 2010, HIMSS published a white paper on meaningful use related to health information exchanges. The white paper provided a summary of Stage 1 meaningful use standards (see Table 5-1).

ELIGIBLE PROFESSIONAL UNDER MEDICARE

This chapter encompasses a lot of discussion about requirements for being an eligible professional (EP). Knowing these requirements is key for qualifying for incentive payments. There are some differences in requirements between Medicare and Medicaid. CMS' EHR Incentive Program website describes eligibility for Medicare as the following:

The Medicare EHR incentive program for eligible professionals (EPs) starts in 2011 and continues through 2016. Eligible professionals can participate for five years throughout the duration of the program. The last year to begin participation is 2014.

The incentives are based on individual providers. Therefore, if you are part of a practice, each eligible professional may qualify for an incentive payment provided they successfully demonstrate meaningful use. Each EP is only eligible for one incentive payment each year, regardless of the number of practices or locations at which they provide services.

Eligibility for Medicare EHR Incentive Program – Eligible Professionals (EPs)
Under the Medicare EHR Incentive Program, EPs must be one of the following:
- Doctors of Medicine or Osteopathy
- Doctors of Dental Surgery or Dental Medicine
- Doctors of Podiatric Medicine
- Doctors of Optometry
- Chiropractors

Physicians who are also eligible as a Medicaid EP must choose between the Medicare and Medicaid incentive programs when they register. Not sure which program to register for? Find more information in the tab marked "Eligibility" on the CMS EHR Incentive Programs website.[1]

NOTE: Medicare EPs may not be hospital-based. An EP is considered hospital-based if 90% or more of the EP's services are performed in a hospital inpatient or

Stage One Objective	Stage One Description	Stage One Measurements
CPOE (Computerized Practitioner Order Entry)	Use CPOE for medication orders directly entered by any licensed healthcare professional who can enter orders into the medical record per state, local and professional guidelines.	More than 30% of unique patients with at least one medication in their medication list seen by the EP or admitted to the eligible hospital or CAH* have at least one medication entered using CPOE.
Drug Screening	Implement drug-drug and drug-allergy interaction checks.	The EP/eligible hospital/CAH has enabled this functionality for the entire EHR reporting period.
Electronic Prescribing	**EP Only:** Generate and transmit permissible prescriptions electronically (eRx).	More than 40% of all permissible prescriptions written by the EP are transmitted electronically using certified EHR technology.
Demographics Recording	Record demographics: preferred language, gender, race, ethnicity, date of birth, and date and preliminary cause of death in the event of mortality in the eligible hospital or CAH.	More than 50% of all unique patients seen by the EP or admitted to the eligible hospital or CAH have demographics as recorded structured data.
Problem List	Maintain up-to-date problem list of current and active diagnoses.	More than 80% of all unique patients seen by the EP or admitted to the eligible hospital or CAH have at least one entry or an indication that no problems are known for the patient recorded as structured data.

*****CAH:** Critical access hospital

Table 5-1: Summary of Stage 1 Meaningful Use Standards

Stage One Objective	Stage One Description	Stage One Measurements
Active Medication List	Maintain active medication list.	More than 80% of all unique patients seen by the EP or admitted to the eligible hospital or CAH have at least one entry (or an indication that the patient is not currently prescribed any medication) recorded as structured data.
Active Medication Allergy List	Maintain active medication allergy list.	More than 80% of all unique patients seen by the EP or admitted to the eligible hospital or CAH have at least one entry (or an indication that the patient has no known medication allergies) recorded as structured data.
Vital Signs	Record and chart vital signs: height, weight, blood pressure, calculate and display BMI, plot and display growth charts for children 2–20 years, including BMI.	For more than 50% of all unique patients age 2 and over seen by the EP or admitted to the eligible hospital or CAH, height, weight, and blood pressure are recorded as structured data.
Smoking Status	Record smoking status for patients 13 years old or older.	More than 50% of all unique patients 13 years or older seen by the EP or admitted to the eligible hospital or CAH have smoking status recorded as structured data.
Clinical Decision Support Rules	Implement one clinical decision support rule and the ability to track compliance with the rule.	Implement one clinical decision support rule.

Table 5-1: *(Continued)*

Stage One Objective	Stage One Description	Stage One Measurements
Clinical Quality Measures Reporting	Report clinical quality measures to CMS or the state.	For 2011, provide aggregate numerator, denominator and exclusions through attestation; for 2012, electronically submit clinical quality measures.
Electronic Copies of Patient Health Information	Provide patients with an electronic copy of their health information (including diagnostic test results, problem list, medication lists, medication allergies, discharge summary, procedures), upon request.	More than 50% of all unique patients of the EP, eligible hospital or CAH who request an electronic copy of their health information are provided with it within three business days.
Hospital Discharge Instructions	**Hospitals Only:** Provide patients with an electronic copy of their discharge instructions at time of discharge, upon request.	More than 50% of all patients who are discharged from an eligible hospital or CAH who request an electronic copy of their discharge instructions are provided with it.
Clinical Summaries	**EPs Only:** Provide clinical summaries for each office visit.	Clinical summaries provided to patients for more than 50% of all office visits within three business days.
One Test of Clinical Information Exchange	Capability to exchange key clinical information (ex: problem list, medication list, medication allergies, diagnostic test results) among providers of care and patient authorized entities electronically.	Performed at least one test of the certified EHR technology's capacity to electronically exchange key clinical information.

Table 5-1: *(Continued)*

Stage One Objective	Stage One Description	Stage One Measurements
Data Protection	Protect electronic health information created or maintained by certified EHR technology through the implementation of appropriate technical capabilities.	Conduct or review a security risk analysis per 45 CFR 164.308(a)(1) and implement updates as necessary and correct identified security deficiencies as part of the EP's, eligible hospital's or CAH's risk management process.
Drug Formulary	Implement drug-formulary checks.	The EP/eligible hospital/CAH has enabled this functionality and has access to at least one internal or external drug formulary for the entire EHR reporting period.
Advance Directives	**Hospitals Only:** Record advance directives for patients 65 years old or older.	More than 50% of all unique patients 65 years old or older admitted to the eligible hospital or CAH have an indication of an advance directive status recorded.
Lab Results	Incorporate clinical lab test results into certified EHR technology as structured data.	More than 40% of all clinical lab test results ordered by the EP, or an authorized provider of the eligible hospital or CAH, for patients admitted during the EHR reporting period whose results are either in a positive/negative or numerical format are incorporated in certified EHR technology as structured data.

Table 5-1: *(Continued)*

Stage One Objective	Stage One Description	Stage One Measurements
Patient Lists	Generate lists of patients by specific conditions to use for quality improvement, reduction of disparities, research or outreach.	Generate at least one report listing patients of the EP, eligible hospital or CAH with a specific condition.
Patient Reminders	**EPs Only:** Send reminders to patients per patient preference for preventive/follow-up care.	More than 20% of all unique patients 65 years or older or 5 years old or younger were sent an appropriate reminder during the EHR reporting period.
Patient Access	**EPs Only:** Provide patients with timely electronic access to their health information (including lab results, problem list, medication lists, medication allergies) within four business days of the information being available to the EP.	More than 10% of all unique patients seen by the EP are provided with timely (available to the patient within four business days of being updated in the certified EHR technology) electronic access to their health information subject to the EP's discretion to withhold certain information.
Patient Education Resources	Use certified EHR technology to identify patient-specific education resources and provide those resources to the patient, if appropriate.	More than 10% of all unique patients seen by the EP or admitted to the eligible hospital or CAH are provided with patient-specific education resources.
Medication Reconciliation	The EP, eligible hospital or CAH who receives a patient from another setting of care or provider of care or believes an encounter is relevant should perform medication reconciliation.	The EP, eligible hospital or CAH performs medication reconciliation for more than 50% of transitions of care in which the patient is transitioned into the care of the EP or admitted to the eligible hospital or CAH.

Table 5-1: *(Continued)*

Stage One Objective	Stage One Description	Stage One Measurements
Care Summary Record Exchange Across Providers	The EP, eligible hospital or CAH who receives a patient from another setting of care or provider of care or refers their patient to another provider of care should provide a summary of care record for each transition of care or referral.	The EP, eligible hospital or CAH who transitions or refers their patient to another setting of care or provider of care provides a summary of care record for more than 50% of transitions of care and referrals.
Immunization	Capability to submit electronic data to immunization registries or Immunization Information Systems and actual submission in accordance with applicable law and practice must be demonstrated.	Perform at least one test of the certified EHR technology's capacity to submit electronic data to immunization registries and follow-up submission if the test is successful (unless none of the immunization registries to which the EP, eligible hospital or CAH submits such information have the capacity to receive such information electronically).
Lab Results	**Hospitals Only:** Capability to submit electronic data on reportable (as required by state or local law) lab results to public health agencies and actual submission in accordance with applicable law and practice must be demonstrated.	Perform at least one test of certified EHR technology's capacity to provide submission of reportable lab results to public health agencies and follow-up submission if the test is successful (unless none of the public health agencies to which the EP, eligible hospital or CAH submits such information have the capacity to receive such information electronically).

Table 5-1: *(Continued)*

Stage One Objective	Stage One Description	Stage One Measurements
Syndromic Surveillance	Capability to submit electronic syndromic surveillance data to public health agencies and actual submission in accordance with applicable law and practice.	Perform at least one test of certified EHR technology's capacity to provide electronic syndromic surveillance data to public health agencies and follow-up submission if the test is successful (unless none of the public health agencies to which the EP, eligible hospital or CAH submits such information have the capacity to receive such information electronically).

Source: HIE Implications in Meaningful Use Stage 1 Requirements, November 2010. Available at www.himss.org/content/files/MU_HIE_Matrix.pdf.

Table 5-1: *(Continued)*

emergency room setting. An EP who is employed by the hospital but performs his or her services in an ambulatory setting is NOT considered hospital based. Examples of hospital-based physicians include a radiologist, anesthesiologist and emergency room physician.

COMBINING EHR INCENTIVE PROGRAMS

The EHR stimulus program is new and it is separate from other active CMS incentive programs, such as the Physicians Quality Reporting Initiative (PQRI) and e-Prescribing. However, if you participate in the EHR incentive program, you cannot receive incentive payments in the e-Prescribing program in the same year. Participating in PQRI and EHR incentives can be combined.

If you are only going to participate in the e-Prescribing incentive program, it is important to note that it is based on allowable submitted charges during the reporting period, while the EHR incentive program provides a determined incentive payment if the requirements of the program are met. In other words, it is volume based, whereas the EHR incentive program is a fixed amount.

As noted above, physicians can participate in PQRI at the same time as the Medicare and Medicaid EHR Incentive Programs.

RECEIVING PAYMENTS

Starting in 2011, meaningful EHR users who use certified EHR technology can receive up to $44,000 over five years under the Medicare incentive program. Incentive payments are made based on the calendar year. To get the maximum incentive payment, Medicare eligible professionals must begin participation by 2012. Table 5-2 illustrates how the payments are distributed:[1]

Important—Any eligible professional participating in any Medicare program who has not adopted a certified EHR by 2015 will have a penalty imposed in the form of a payment reduction to their Medicare reimbursement. The reduction starts at one percent and increases up to five percent for every year that a Medicare eligible professional does not demonstrate meaningful use.

More information about the incentive payout and penalties for not adopting can be found the CMS website.[1]

Payment Amounts	Medicare EP Qualifies to Receive First Payment in 2011	Medicare EP Qualifies to Receive First Payment in 2012	Medicare EP Qualifies to Receive First Payment in 2013	Medicare EP Qualifies to Receive First Payment in 2014	Medicare EP Qualifies to Receive First Payment in 2015
Payment Amount for 2011	$18,000.00	$0.00	$0.00	$0.00	$0.00
Payment Amount for 2012	$12,000.00	$18,000.00	$0.00	$0.00	$0.00
Payment Amount for 2013	$8,000.00	$12,000.00	$15,000.00	$0.00	$0.00
Payment Amount for 2014	$4,000.00	$8,000.00	$12,000.00	$12,000.00	$0.00
Payment Amount for 2015	$2,000.00	$4,000.00	$8,000.00	$8,000.00	$0.00
Payment Amount for 2016	$0.00	$2,000.00	$4,000.00	$4,000.00	$0.00
TOTAL Payment Amount	$44,000.00	$44,000.00	$39,000.00	$24,000.00	$0.00

Table 5-2: Payment Distribution

ELIGIBLE PROFESSIONAL UNDER MEDICAID

As noted previously, an EP can participate in either Medicare or Medicaid. Accordingly, the EP requirements are different under Medicaid, which is defined as the following by CMS:

> The Medicaid EHR incentive program is voluntarily offered and administered by States and territories. States can start offering their program to eligible professionals (EPs) as early as 2011. The program continues through 2021. EPs can participate for 6 years throughout the duration of the program. The last year to begin participation is 2016.
>
> The incentives are based on the individual providers. Therefore, if you are part of a practice, each eligible professional may qualify for an incentive payment provided they meet the requirements for the program. Each EP is only eligible for one incentive payment each year, regardless of how many practices or locations they provide services.
>
> ### Eligibility for Medicaid EHR Incentive Program – Eligible Professionals (EPs)
>
> Under the Medicaid EHR incentive program, EPs include the following:
> - Physicians (Pediatricians have special eligibility and payment rules)
> - Nurse Practitioners (NPs)
> - Certified Nurse-Midwives (CNMs)
> - Dentists
> - Physician Assistants (PAs) who provide services in a Federally Qualified Health Center (FQHC) or rural health clinic (RHC) that is led by a PA
>
> Medicaid eligible professionals must also meet patient volume criteria, providing services to those attributable to Medicaid or, in some cases, needy individuals. To see if you may be eligible, click on the tab marked "Eligibility" on the CMS EHR Incentive Programs website.[1]

NOTE: Similar to Medicare, any Medicaid eligible professionals who are hospital-based, performing 90 percent or more of his or her services in a hospital inpatient or emergency room setting, may not participate. The reason for this is because the hospital is likely getting paid to participate; therefore, funds have already been designated for the hospital. Also, as with Medicare, the EP can still participate in PQRI but cannot participate in E-prescribing and EHR incentives at the same time.

MEDICAID INCENTIVE PAYMENTS

The Medicaid incentive payments differ significantly from Medicare and so do the qualifications. To qualify for Medicaid incentive payments, Medicaid eligible professionals must *adopt, implement, upgrade or demonstrate meaningful use of certified EHR technology in the first year of participation*. Under Medicaid, the EP can be eligible for the first year just by adopting or upgrading an existing system and does not have to be a meaningful user initially. This is allowed because it is assumed the organization that provides services to Medicaid patients requires more up-front financial assistance.

However, to receive additional funding, the Medicaid EPs must demonstrate meaningful use in years 2–6 of participation. For calendar years 2011–2021, participants can receive up to $63,750 over 6 years under the Medicaid EHR incentive program.

Each state is responsible for funding the incentive payments under Medicaid. Table 5-3 shows the payout schedule.[1]

Important—Similar to Medicare, EPs that do not adopt a certified EHR will have their Medicaid reimbursement reduced by one percent starting in 2015.

STATE SPECIFIC INFORMATION

Under the HITECH Act, each state is given the option to voluntarily offer the Medicaid incentive program to their eligible Medicaid professionals. The CMS EHR Incentive Programs website provides information that may be state specific, including grants and other incentives that may be localized. These additional programs fall under the title "A Health Information Technology Planning Advance Planning Document (HIT PAPD)," which is a plan of action that requests federal matching funds and approval to accomplish the planning necessary for a state agency to determine the need for and plan the acquisition of health IT equipment, services, or both. As a result, there may be additional incentives or federally funded programs. For example, some states have been given grants to expand Internet access in rural areas.

Also, CMS frequently engages in state-specific outreach activities to educate the states on the Medicaid EHR Incentive Program and to gather feedback from the states about the program. Information on state-specific activities can be found at the CMS EHR Incentive Programs website.[1]

REASONS FOR NOT PARTICIPATING

There are some legitimate reasons why participating in EHR incentives may not be right for your practice. Certain specialties, such as pediatrics or plastic surgeons, generally do not see enough Medicare or Medicaid patients to qualify. You may also be nearing retirement or hoping your practice will be acquired by the hospital. Therefore, the cost to purchase the system may not be justified. Also, there are situations in which a provider is not ready for an EHR or they feel like there is no EHR qualified for their specialty or to meet their needs. Some will even argue that incentive money is just a pass-through to the vendors and the physician never benefits. However, when compared to self-financing, it is certainly a benefit to have the incentive to help offset the cost.

Physicians that are high producers in terms of patient volume will often argue that slowing them down is more costly and outweighs any one-time incentive payment. While there could be some truth to this, over time, this thinking would likely reverse once penalties kick in, assuming the practice has a significant amount of Medicare patients. It is also common for commercial payers to follow Medicare guidelines so other payers may eventually consider similar penalties. While there could be myriad reasons for not participating, most experts will agree it is not a matter of "if", it is now a matter of "when." The only exception to this would be in circumstances where there are significant threats to a successful outcome, such as moving forward with an EHR that is no longer supported or where there is significant opposition to adoption.

	Medicaid EP Qualifies to Receive First Payment in 2011	Medicaid EP Qualifies to Receive First Payment in 2012	Medicaid EP Qualifies to Receive First Payment in 2013	Medicaid EP Qualifies to Receive First Payment in 2014	Medicaid EP Qualifies to Receive First Payment in 2015	Medicaid EP Qualifies to Receive First Payment in 2016
Payment Amount in 2011	$21,250.00	$0.00	$0.00	$0.00	$0.00	$0.00
Payment Amount in 2012	$8,500.00	$21,250.00	$0.00	$0.00	$0.00	$0.00
Payment Amount in 2013	$8,500.00	$8,500.00	$21,250.00	$0.00	$0.00	$0.00
Payment Amount in 2014	$8,500.00	$8,500.00	$8,500.00	$21,250.00	$0.00	$0.00
Payment Amount in 2015	$8,500.00	$8,500.00	$8,500.00	$8,500.00	$21,250.00	$0.00
Payment Amount in 2016	$8,500.00	$8,500.00	$8,500.00	$8,500.00	$8,500.00	$21,250.00
Payment Amount in 2017	$0.00	$8,500.00	$8,500.00	$8,500.00	$8,500.00	$8,500.00
Payment Amount in 2018	$0.00	$0.00	$8,500.00	$8,500.00	$8,500.00	$8,500.00
Payment Amount in 2019	$0.00	$0.00	$0.00	$8,500.00	$8,500.00	$8,500.00
Payment Amount in 2020	$0.00	$0.00	$0.00	$0.00	$8,500.00	$8,500.00
Payment Amount in 2021	$0.00	$0.00	$0.00	$0.00	$0.00	$8,500.00
TOTAL Incentive Payments	$63,750.00	$63,750.00	$63,750.00	$63,750.00	$63,750.00	$63,750.00

Table 5-3: Payout Schedule

FUTURE UPDATES AND STAYING CURRENT

The official CMS EHR Incentive Programs website is updated frequently; however, it is not 100 percent provider specific and finding answers can be difficult. Several websites, including HIMSS' (www.himss.org), monitor and publish updates in a summary format. Other healthcare associations, such as the American Association of Family Physicians (AAFP) and the American Medical Association (AMA) also provide frequent, easy-to-read-and-understand summary updates.

Vendors can also be resourceful. However, be cautious of vendors providing information designed to pressure you into purchasing an EHR. For example, vendors will often use the "fear of loss" tactic as way to rush a decision by implying the funding will run out or they will not have time to get your system installed to participate in the maximum amount. There are also vendors who will advocate not participating in EHR incentives over fears that the government is trying to control your practice or use your data to pursue you. These are usually vendors that are not qualified as a certified vendor, and they feel threatened by the imposed requirements. Obviously, any provider that participates in Medicare has to provide information to the government, so this argument is irrelevant.

CONCLUSION

It is important to emphasize that coverage of the HITECH Act provided in this chapter only includes a small subset of the Act's content and is mostly relevant to the adoption of EHRs. Other resources and information concerning the HITECH Act can be found at www.cms.gov and at ONC's primary site at www.healthit.hhs.gov. The main purpose of this chapter is to highlight the primary parts of the Act that apply to financial incentives for adopting EHRs. The Act also covers policies related to HIPAA and new Security Rules.

Providers treating Medicare or Medicaid patients that want to receive the benefit of incentives, or at a minimum, seek to avoid any subsequent penalties, appear to have little choice other than to adopt an EHR. In summary, virtually all of the financial benefits are time sensitive, with a diminishing rate of return for late adopters. Starting early will help ensure maximum benefits are obtainable.

REFERENCE

1.   The Official Website for the Medicare and Medicaid Electronic Health Records (EHR) Incentive Programs. http://www.cms.gov/EHrIncentivePrograms/. Accessed December 10, 2011.

CHAPTER 6

Vendor Vetting

INTRODUCTION

Vendor vetting is the most critical part of the electronic health record (EHR) adoption process. Selecting the wrong vendor can have devastating consequences. With hundreds of EHR vendors in the marketplace today, it is common to feel overwhelmed by the choices that are available. Many physicians feel a great deal of anxiety about choosing the "right" vendor and the "right" product. This chapter will help you in navigating this process.

It been well documented that 30 percent of all EHRs purchased will never be fully installed. Even more disturbing, however, is the fact that, of the systems that are installed, many are never fully used. According to a recent CDC study, only 4 percent of EHRs are fully used at the point of care.[1]

Following a proven process for success can help a practice avoid adding itself to these statistics or having to uninstall an EHR and resume work with paper records. Although many processes for selecting vendors have been developed through the years, it is easy to get off track because of the amount of work that is often required by the adoption process. In addition, trying to complete this process without any guidance can be extremely overwhelming.

For starters, the critical success factors to selecting a good vendor are as follows:

- **Use a structured process.** Have a "flight plan" to know where you are going or where you want to go. Creating a structured EHR adoption process should include assembling a vendor selection committee from a small group of staff members, creating a list of project goals and objectives, and coming up with a short list of vendors to review. You might also create an EHR mission statement or draft a list of guiding principles.
- **Define practice needs beforehand.** Create a list of requirements and identify any special needs your practice may have. For example, if your practice has several remote locations, you will want to find out how vendors can connect these offices together. If the practice provides occupational health services or operates as a rural health clinic, there may be special billing and reporting requirements that need to be addressed. Having a list of these special requirements prepared will help you make apples-to-apples comparisons as you look

at different EHR systems. Start by writing down the top ten functions the practice must have. You can also create a list of desired or preferred functions. Compare these functions to your mission statement to make sure you are staying on course. Try not to dream up the "perfect" system; perfect systems do not exist. Rather, begin by defining your practice's basic requirements—those that are most critical to your organization.

- **Create tools to assist you in decision making.** After defining your needs, use this information to create your own vendor selection tools. For example, convert your top ten requirements into a product demonstration scorecard. Create a ranking system to score how well each vendor meets each requirement. Include room on the scorecard for your comments about what you liked and did not like during the demonstration. You might also consider creating a demonstration script for each vendor to follow. This script describes a patient visit scenario and it allows vendors to demonstrate how their products address the scenario. Usually, vendors will come prepared to demonstrate a well-rehearsed scenario that is specifically designed to make their product look good. Using the same script for each vendor allows you to compare each product on a level playing field. Appendix A provides more suggestions for creating decision-making tools and includes templates for scorecards and demonstration scripts.

- **Develop a request for proposal.** Although developing a request for proposal (RFP) can be a time-consuming task, it is an essential tool for evaluating potential vendors. An RFP provides vendors with information about your practice and provides the first formal documentation of your expectations for a project. The vendor responses will allow for side-by-side comparison of products. Because responding to a well-prepared RFP takes a fair amount of effort on the vendor's part, invite only serious contenders to provide your practice with a proposal. A sample RFP is provided in Appendix A.

- **Make sure you include key users in the vendor selection process.** Allowing staff members to participate in this process will create a multitude of benefits. For starters, as subject matter experts on the practice's workflow, they bring valuable experience to bear in this process. They can best determine if the product will solve or create problems. Including them in the process also encourages full adoption because they will develop a sense of ownership and responsibility for decisions relating to the system. It is also a good practice to have several sets of eyes review a big project like this one, just in case something is missed. Working through the selection process alone is never recommended; plus, you will have no one else to share the blame if it does turn out to be a bad decision.

- **Prepare for the product demonstration.** Vendors will typically come on site to demonstrate their software. When possible, it is best to schedule the demonstrations after hours or late in the afternoon when there are fewer distractions. This is not something to you should attempt to fit into a lunch break. Keep in mind that the demonstration is only one step in a long process. It is common for preferred vendors to come back for a second and third demonstration before a final decision is made. Sometimes it is best to invite only a few people to the first round of demonstrations so that you can narrow the field down to two vendors. The sooner you can narrow the field, the easier the selection process becomes. Often vendors can provide demonstrations via the Internet using tools like WebEx or GoToMyPC. Here is a list of tips and suggestions to help you prepare for demonstrations.

1. Use a room that is large enough for everyone to fit into and that allows vendors to set up their equipment easily. Vendors may also bring extra staff with them to assist during demonstrations. Sometimes the best option is to use the waiting room after hours. If you are planning to look at several vendors in one day, you may want to consider using a meeting room at a local hospital or hotel. Going off site may help minimize distractions.

2. Plan on spending two hours per vendor demonstration.

3. Request that the vendors deliver their demonstrations in a sequence that is consistent with basic patient flow through your practice. For example, to fully appreciate the system's ability to manage the entire workflow, ask the vendor to demonstrate the product showing the workflow from the beginning to the end of a typical patient visit. A fully integrated system should be capable of demonstrating this sequence without toggling between applications. It is best to observe this process without interruptions so that you can evaluate the efficiencies of each system. You can later go back and ask questions or drill down into each phase of the workflow.

4. Try to minimize distractions during the demonstration by asking everyone to turn off their cell phones and not bring their laptop computers.

5. Be sure to schedule the demonstration on a day when the right people are available to participate.

6. Use your scorecard and other system evaluation tools. Require vendors to show you what they are describing. Vendors are often very comfortable describing how functions work, but it is important for you to actually see the EHR in action.

7. Stay on time and make sure each vendor receives equal time to present. Again, two hours is recommended per vendor.

8. Do not be afraid to ask the vendor to hand over the controls to allow you to drive the system. In some cases, a vendor will leave a trial version of their software to allow staff extra time to play with the system.

9. Consider asking vendors to do a demonstration in an examination room. Have a staff member stage a mock patient visit with the vendor serving as EHR scribe while a provider from your practice does a mock examination using the EHR. This "hands-on" activity will illuminate how the product actually works at the point of care by creating a real-world scenario.

10. Although it is important to see the entire system at work and vendors are usually very good at doing so, it is common for some features to be considered add-on modules. Be sure to tell vendors that they must make you aware of any features they demonstrate that are not included in the core system. Common add-on modules usually include document imaging, handheld charge capturing, reporting tools, patient portals, electronic data

services, and eligibility. Most practices today are looking at fully integrated solutions that include all the modules and features. However, we caution that you not assume all features are included in the base system. Vendors generally give a larger discount when practices bundle all of the add-on modules. However, we recommend that you pay for add-on modules only on activation. For example, if you are buying a fully integrated solution, you would likely install the practice management system first. Therefore, payment for modules that apply only to the EHR system should be deferred until those add-on modules are activated and ready for use. Paying for full activation of all features at the beginning of the install is not recommended.

- **Be aware of deceptive features.** One of the features of an EHR system that is often misleading is the ability of a provider to click and point his/her way through an examination. Although such features do exist—and, of course, the program worked flawlessly during the sales presentation—what happens when the provider clicks through all the options yet still has more to say? Is the provider expected to key in the remainder of his/her comments? Is there even a space available in the form for this information?

Some EHR vendors would have you believe that every office visit will fit nicely and neatly into the system template. Our experience has been that templates will take you only so far before an alternative means of documentation is necessary. For example, a common problem for providers when working with EHRs is how to handle the "Oh, Doc. By the way…" moment that often occurs at the end of an examination. You have closed out the patient's EHR, shaken his hand, and are reaching for the door. "Oh, Doctor. By the way, my left knee has also been hurting." Now, what are you going to do? How are you going to document this second problem using a template for the first problem, which is high blood pressure? In the past, you would have just made a quick note in the record or an addendum to your dictation. With EHRs, it would be time-prohibitive to open another template for left knee pain or attempt to go back and point and click your way through another clinical pathway. Moreover, you are not going to have a template for every problem. This scenario brings us to the most important feature of any EHR system, charting by exception, which is described below.

Successful EHR solutions all have one thing in common—it is called *flexible charting* or *charting by exception*. If an exceptional situation crops up, a good EHR system allows providers to adapt "on the fly." There should be more than one option for inputting data. Providers can choose from voice recognition, dictation, handwriting, or physically keying in physician notes. However, not all EHR systems provide this type of flexibility on the fly. Physicians can get stuck without an easy way to input information, which indeed forces them into the role of data-entry clerks—not a good use of physician time. Lack of system flexibility of this kind readily leads to frustration, and it is the leading cause when a practice chooses to uninstall its EHR system.

In light of the need for flexibility, during the vendor demonstration, be sure to evaluate the system's ability to handle unusual documenting scenarios. You must assess how the system accommodates workflow deviations. Attempting to capture absolutely everything in a structured format simply is not feasible—nor is it a reasonable expectation. Nevertheless, many EHR systems do not allow providers sufficient flexibility to accommodate real-world clinical situations. Although it is necessary to enter patient data into structured data fields to ensure accurate reporting, full Medicare reimbursement, and stimulus eligibility under the American Recovery and Reinvestment Act of 2009, practices should look beyond using EHRs as mere databases when they have the opportunity to use them for practice transformation.

CLINICAL CONTENT

Another pitfall in vendor selection is the availability of clinical content. Often EHR vendors will leave the development of clinical content up to the providers under the assumption that each physician will want to design clinical pathways around his/her own preferences. Although this approach sounds reasonable, consider how impractical it would be to program a database for each physician's unique clinical style. For example, take a problem like a stomachache. Are you going to call it a "stomachache" or possibly "abdominal pain," "acute abdomen," "stomach pain," or "belly ache"? If you call it "abdominal pain," but later conduct a search for it under another name, you will not be able to locate data for which you are looking.

Because of this challenge, some organizations have adopted national standardized databases such as the Systematized Nomenclature of Medicine–Clinical Terms (SNOMED CT) or the International Classification of Diseases, Ninth Revision (ICD-9) as guidelines for what medical terminology to use. Adapting to a standardized database can be challenging for physicians, especially given the wealth of synonyms in medical terminology. Take pharmaceuticals, for example; the same medication can be referred to by its generic name, multiple brand names, or clinical name. Although some EHR systems have features that allow for slang searches, the results are mapped only to the clinical name or to the standardized reference. Nonetheless, clinical content is a feature that must be embedded in the system; otherwise, undertaking this development function (or agreeing to take it on) will be an overwhelming, time-consuming and ongoing task. It has been our experience that paucity in clinical content is a major cause for EHR failure. Vendors who do not offer clinical content will often promote their system as an "opportunity" (for you, or them—with additional fees) to design and customize the EHR around your practice's unique style. This approach is very misleading, however, and it is virtually impossible to achieve satisfactory results for the system within a reasonable amount of time and with minimal disruption to the practice because of the complexities involved in developing this content.

In addition, please note that vendors who provide integrated practice management systems must conform to the coding standards of International Classification of Diseases, Tenth Revision (www.cms.gov/ICD10/), by October 1, 2013.

SITE VISIT

Peer-to-Peer Site Visit

A site visit to a practice using the EHR you are considering is one of the final steps in the system selection process and it is one of the most important steps. Visiting other organizations that have already installed and worked with your EHR finalist allows you to observe your vendor in a "real world" setting. In addition, you will get an opportunity to visit a practice similar to yours that has successfully undergone the transformation. A site visit can offer many benefits, including receiving valuable advice on what not to do.

Selecting the right site to visit is very important. Although some may argue that the ideal location for a site visit is anywhere in Hawaii, organizations should select a site that is similar in size and structure to their own.

Members of the selection committee should try to visit a practice in the same geographic region whenever possible. Aside from reducing travel costs, this approach allows you to ask colleagues what they really think of the vendor's regional support team.

In most cases, vendors will provide you with a choice of at least two sites to visit. They may try to steer you to one particular site—commonly known as the "showcase site"—which often receives special favors in exchange for the inconvenience of frequent visitors.

Ask if the vendor compensates the site visit host. Some hosts receive kickbacks for helping the vendor promote their system to potential buyers. Some practices are used extensively for site visits and are coached by the vendor for success.

In some cases, host sites are directly managed by a vendor's IT department. If so, assume allegiance. Also pay close attention to the number of staff members required to support the system at the host sites. Vendors may promise to reduce your need for medical records staff. However, if the new system causes you to hire three new system programmers, the trade-off was clearly not worth it.

Showcase sites should be viewed with a cautious eye. You may go to a regional user group meeting later only to find out that the host site's wonderful experiences with the system are an exception to the rule. That being said, showcase sites should not be avoided entirely. It can be an educational experience to see how the software is being used to its maximum potential. However, if you do go to a showcase site, make sure you also visit an average site.

Site visits can be expensive—especially if the site is not within driving distance. However, travel expenses often can be negotiated with vendors. Although some vendors will offer to pay all related travel expenses for the site visit team, others will agree to pay half of these expenses. Final arrangements are likely dependent on internal company policies for the vendor and potential buyer.

However, we offer a word of caution regarding accepting expensive hotel rooms and lavish meals from vendors. You do not want the committee to evaluate a system that everyone will work with day in and day out based on how great a time they had on that two-day road trip.

When talking to users at the site visit, it is important to pay attention to body language, observe facial expressions, and listen for mixed messages, cynical comments, and guarded language. Do not be afraid to ask follow-up questions if users appear to be withholding information. If the vendor is present, ask if you can have a private moment with the users. Sometimes it can be intimidating for customers to give honest answers in front of their sales representatives.

Also look for more subtle clues about the system. Do users have a lot of cheat sheets and sticky notes on their monitors? If so, these may be signs that the system is not designed for intuitive use and that it requires users to memorize a lot of codes and keyboard strokes to navigate through the forms.

Also, be sure to watch for the basic response time of the screens. Observe the system's general responsiveness when files are opened and saved (e.g., scanned images). A site visit is conducted in a live environment with active users and transactions under way. Slowness in systems is not always caused by the software, however. System speed is usually influenced by hardware and network configurations. If the system seems slow, ask for an explanation.

Using an interview guide will help you ensure that all your questions are addressed. After you return to your practice, these notes will help you better recall your impression of the site. A sample site visit interview guide/checklist is provided in Appendix A. After the site visit, the evaluation committee should regroup to discuss findings and impressions either at the end of the day or immediately the next day. If the group waits two weeks to get together to compare notes, valuable information will be lost—especially if another site visit is held in the intervening time. One person on the evaluation committee should have the responsibility of managing the site visit interview guide/checklist and sharing a summary report with members of the site visit team and members of the selection committee who were not present for the site visit.

Corporate Site Visit

It is valuable to inspect the corporate headquarters of the prospective vendor. This site visit will ensure that your practice is not buying a system from a vendor who is operating out of a garage. A corporate site visit should include the following:

- Corporate overview
- Introductions to senior leadership
- Review of implementation methodologies and professional services
- An overview of their technology roadmap and their vision for the future
- Introductions to those who are responsible for supporting the system and a thorough explanation of their policies and procedures for providing support
- Tour of the facility, development department, and data center
- Additional product demonstrations
- Inspection of special features
- Client success stories and benchmarks for the return on investment
- Contracting expectations and financing options (payment terms)

- Review of vendor financial records for solvency.
  - If the organization is a publicly held company, this data is available as a public record. Private companies may require a nondisclosure agreement before they will share/release financial information. Avoid transactions with vendors that prohibit access to their financial records.
  - Information on the number of years in business and the number of systems sold should also be acquired.
- Wrap-up and review of next steps.

REFERENCE CHECKS

At this stage in the vetting process, you are likely ready to make your vendor choice. At the same time, you are feeling very exhausted and are ready to move into the next phase of the project, which is contract negotiations. However, reference checks are extremely important. They allow you an opportunity to gather a wide sampling on user satisfaction. It is not uncommon to hear some complaints during reference calls. Keep in mind that not all complaints are the vendor's fault. Look for a pattern in responses. If several customers complain about slow response time for support, this is not an isolated problem. If only one person has this complaint, it could have just been an off-day for the vendor. Here is a list of topics and questions you should consider addressing when making reference calls:

- Why they selected the software
- How they compare system performance versus expectations
- The quality of training provided
- How the implementation team performs
- Their ability to meet schedules and deadlines
- The attitude demonstrated by the vendor staff (friendly, adversarial, etc.)
- How problems during implementation are handled and resolved
- How bugs are handled
- How unexpected requests, such as change in scope, are handled
- How the vendor assists with the change management aspects of implementation
- How upgrades and new releases are handled
- Unexpected surprises (good and bad):
  - Challenge of finding and retaining IT talent to support the system
  - Major benefits of the system
  - Major limitations of the system
  - System outages vis-à-vis contingency planning and restoration processes
  - Vendor responsiveness to support and maintenance problems
  - Hidden costs
  - Customization issues
  - How did the vendor handle the difficulties?
  - Did the vendor try to blame others or take responsibility themselves?
  - Does the vendor have a user group association or a way for customers to network with other users?

When possible, use open-ended questions so respondents have the opportunity to provide additional information. Good final questions might be, "If you had to do it over again, would you still choose the same system?" and "Would you recommend the system to a friend?"

CONCLUSION

For motivated buyers, the vendor vetting process typically takes 60 to 90 days. For less motivated buyers and for practices with required special features, this process can take up to one year. Try your best to avoid making the vendor search an exhaustive process that looks at every system on the market. It is best to start with a prescreening process that allows you to narrow down your vendor options to four or five choices. A list of the top 20 most common mistakes practices make when vetting EHR vendors follows:

1. Did not determine practice readiness to adapt to the technology being considered.
2. Did not determine any pre-existing operational compromises.
3. Did not develop diversified EHR workgroups/committees to complete the due diligence process.
4. Did not seek input from industry experts familiar with EHR deployment.
5. Did not build consensus among the entire group.
6. Did not select the vendor based on their ability to meet practice objectives.
7. Did not define the practice objectives to be met.
8. Did not fully research the vendor's capacity to accomplish the objectives.
9. Did not commit the proper resources to research vendors.
10. Did not properly define implementation objectives.
11. Did not establish the proper vendor implementation incentives.
12. Did not establish appropriate levels of vendor accountability.
13. Did not ensure proper practice protection in the vendor contract (see Chapter 8).
14. Did not establish any vendor performance expectations.
15. Did not plan financially for the hard and soft costs of the project.
16. Did not plan financially for the initial decreases in productivity.
17. Did not understand or expect additional fees (e.g., recurring fees, customization fees, interfacing and integrating fees, transaction fees).
18. Did not properly evaluate the technology's practical use in a live setting.
19. Did not properly research the vendor.
20. Did not properly research the integration requirements.

An EHR will touch every part of an ambulatory practice. EHR implementation and optimization are and should be transformational processes. It is critical—particularly for physician owners—to allow those who will be responsible for implementation to guide and lead the process of transformation. Although the focus of this chapter is vendor vetting, technology usage, workflow, content and training must be addressed in each phase of the project to ensure the transformation is complete and the EHR does not become a very expensive, digitized paper record. To be successful with EHRs, physicians and other providers must be willing to submit to the process and allow themselves to be novices again. Everyone should be prepared to keep their eyes wide open during the vendor evaluation process.

REFERENCE

1. EHR failures: can we do better than the average? July 31, 2008. http://www.healthcare-informatics.com/ME2/dirmod.asp?nm=&type=Blog&mod=View+Topic&mid=&tier=7&id=EDE4B65E6FA344C286C02EFB2CD4D223 Accessed January 12, 2011.

CHAPTER 7

Making the Vendor Decision

INTRODUCTION

The previous chapter offered proven processes for evaluating vendors. It did not, however, address the most important part of the process: making a decision. After a thorough vendor vetting initiative, sorting through your options can still be a mind-boggling proposition. Also, constant changes in the market for electronic health records (EHRs) can muddy the waters. Ongoing mergers and acquisitions among vendors add to the confusion, making the path unclear. In addition, there is the added pressure of the knowledge that selecting a vendor can be a career-defining (or career-limiting) decision.

For many practices, the final mile is the most difficult part of the journey. It is not uncommon to undergo a comprehensive vendor vetting process and still be on the fence as to which vendor is best suited for your practice. You may also find that you are experiencing what is sometimes called "analysis paralysis," which is a tongue-in-cheek way of saying that you are second guessing yourself by reexamining all the information collected during the vetting process. You may even get "cold feet" as you start worrying about the costs. You might start to rethink all your research. Again, this response is very common, which is why we have devoted this chapter to assist you in choosing a vendor. Furthermore, this chapter precedes our discussion of strategies for vendor contracting and negotiations; it can be very grueling to enter into contract negotiations with an unqualified vendor or with a vendor who does not ultimately get selected.

After undergoing a thorough vetting process, many practices stall in making a vendor decision. It feels like "the point of no return." It can also be difficult for a practice at this stage to consider excluding a vendor who has been involved in the process for months. Human nature encourages us to feel attached to the sales representative and we may have a sense of obligation toward him/her after establishing a warm relationship during the sales process. To make matters more difficult, other vendors who were included in the process generally start turning up the pressure on the practice to make a decision. In some cases, vendors will start creating incentives to prompt practices to make impulsive decisions. The salesperson is usually getting pressure from his or her boss to close the sale and bring in a signed contract. It is at this point that sales representatives will often introduce some tried-and-true sales tactics to induce a decision. Accordingly, here are some of the most common sales tactics to be aware of:

- **End-of-month, -quarter, or -year special pricing.** This is the most common trick in the book. The vendor will drop the price at "the last minute" and tell you there is an end-of-month, end-of-quarter, or end-of-year special and—to take advantage of this great discount—that it requires a commitment before the discount expires. The intent is to force a decision by imposing an artificial deadline. If a discount can be given today, the vendor should honor it later without using strong-arm tactics.

- **The letter of intent.** The vendor tells you they must get a letter of intent before they can agree to offer discounts. Alternatively, they might tell you that, before they can discuss discounts of any kind, they must have you sign a contract—one that includes an option for you to back out if you cannot agree on terms and pricing. There is absolutely no reason to sign any agreement or contract until you are ready to buy. Vendors may try this approach to this to see if you are a serious buyer or as a way to find out if you are working with more than one vendor.

- **The special showcase site promise.** The vendor offers to make your practice a "special showcase site." Although such sites do exist (see Chapter 6), showcase sites are usually only offered by start-up vendors. If this option is offered, the vendor will generally compensate the showcase site or they will provide special concessions as a way of making the practice successful.

- **The corporate retreat.** Vendors will sometimes offer a paid trip to attend a swanky corporate retreat. Although this offer can be extremely tempting, the intent is to put you through a sales process similar to the well-known 90-minute timeshare presentation. The vendor tries to make you feel obligated to purchase their product/service because they provided you with a paid trip.

- **Gifts and special favors.** Accepting a gift valued at more than $25 from any vendor is never recommended. Accepting expensive gifts can create a conflict of interest and make a difficult situation for you personally should the vendor decision turn out to be unsatisfactory. Do not allow gifts to tarnish the integrity of the vetting process.

- **Misleading information or embellishment.** Some vendors will make statements that are not entirely accurate to provoke a decision to buy their software. Statements that seem misleading should be verified. Vendors will also drop untruthful information about their competition. A vendor that talks badly about other vendors generally fears losing you as a potential sale and is making a desperate attempt to discourage you from buying the other system.

- **An unrealistic promise.** Vendors will sometimes make commitments and promises knowing that they or their product/service will not meet the requirements. The vendor knows that, once you buy the system, you are virtually 100 percent committed. A broken promise will be disappointing, but the vendor knows it will not be enough to justify returning the system. To reduce the potential impact of unrealistic promises, the vendor should be required to defer a portion of their invoice until they make good on their promises. (In

Chapter 8, we provide additional details on how to avoid the unrealistic promise.)

- **Aggressive statements.** Although rare, some vendors have been known to strong-arm a decision by having you believe that there will not be any room to get you on the training schedule if you delay your decision. They may even suggest there is a government mandate or penalty that will result in a negative impact to the practice if your decision is delayed. They may also suggest an upcoming price increase on the hardware or software as another way of setting an artificial deadline.

Most vendors will use some tactics to make a sale; this approach comes with the territory and it should be expected. Generally, vendors will respect your decision if you tell them you need more time or ask them not to pressure you into making a decision. From our experience, vendors who lead and provide transparent information are far more successful than those who try to use gimmicks or become aggressive.

STEPS FOR MAKING THE VENDOR DECISION

Now that you are aware of common sales tactics, let us examine some options for making your vendor of choice decision so you can start negotiations and contracting:

1. Remind yourself that (1) there is no "perfect" vendor, (2) paper records are also imperfect, and (3) this decision is necessary for the practice to remain viable in the future.
2. Doing nothing is the most expensive option.
3. Consider for a moment just the basics and fundamentals of each vendor option. Although it may sound like we are oversimplifying the decision-making process, over-thinking can sometimes lead to mistakes. Use the decision-making tool illustrated in Table 7-1 to help you sort out your thoughts. It will help you rate each vendor on the top ten things that are most important to the practice.
4. After examining your basic requirements, take a look at some of the deal breakers:
    a. Does the system meet the requirements for practice participation in the incentive program through the American Recovery and Reinvestment Act of 2009 (ARRA)?
    b. How is the system supported?
    c. How are you charged and invoiced for technical support (e.g., hourly, monthly, quarterly, annually, via separate support contract)?
    d. Who will provide your hardware?
    e. Does the system meet your interfacing needs?
    f. Does the system conform to health information exchange requirements?
    g. Does the vendor provide technical support 24 hours a day, 7 days a week?
    h. Are upgrades included in the maintenance fees?
    i. How frequently do system updates take place?
    j. Does the vendor have a training plan and a project plan you can review?
    k. How many installations does the vendor have in your immediate area?
    l. Does the vendor have a testing plan? (Testing the system is necessary to ensure integrity of the data and increase the success of implementation.)

Score Each Vendor on a Scale of 1 to 5			
Requirements	**Vendor A**	**Vendor B**	**Vendor C**
Ease of use			
Meets most of the preferred requirements			
Vendor references			
Site visit experience			
Corporate site visit experience			
Results of demonstration scorecard			
Vendor responsiveness			
Meets compliance standards			
Has local installs			
Has clinical content specific to your specialty			

Table 7-1: Tool for Scoring Vendors

    m. Can the system be implemented in stages and phases? (This allows some budgeting flexibility.)

5. Available financing options are generally also critical to the vendor decision. Some vendors allow a practice to defer payments until the system is installed. Often they will also work with a practice to help spread out payments. Others will offer special financing promotions. Consider the following when making your financing decision:

    a. Identify all costs, including hardware (e.g., scanners, personal computers [PCs], tablet PCs, digital diagnostic equipment), software licensing, installation, training, annual maintenance fees, and support fees. You need to know the cost of installation as well as annual costs associated with product maintenance.

    b. Other costs to consider include network fees and database licenses. Implementation and training fees add up quickly. Remember also to consider travel expenses if the vendor is out of state.

    c. Consider going to your local bank. Sometimes, they will offer the best financing option.

    d. To manage your expenses, consider the following:

        i. Determine a business plan and budget.

        ii. Consider a bank loan. Loans for technology and business equipment usually have three- to five-year terms with favorable interest rates.

        iii. Consider contracting with an application service provider, which can reduce the up-front investment and hardware maintenance costs.

        iv. Do not overbuy or prepay for services that are non-tangible, such as training or consulting fees.

     e. **Important:** Do not allow the vendor to withdraw money from the loan until your bank or leasing company has provided your final loan approval. You should always structure your payment terms based on project milestones and/or accomplishments. Here is an easy granular payment plan to follow:

        i. 25 percent due at signing of the contract

        ii. 25 percent due on successful completion of software and hardware installation

        iii. 25 percent due on successful go-live

        iv. 25 percent due thirty (30) days after go-live

        v. Annual maintenance fees due at go-live

        vi. Professional services and travel costs paid as incurred

6. Review your goals alongside vendor options. Recall all the things you hope to accomplish with an EHR system. Examine how each vendor you are considering will help you meet each of these goals. Would one vendor solve more of your problems than the others would?

7. Review the scores from the request for proposal (RFP) to determine which vendor is willing to tie the RFP to the contract. A vendor who honors their promises will agree to this condition.

8. Consider consulting third-party (unbiased) organizations, such as KLAS (www .klasresearch.com) that monitor and rank vendor performance. When a practice agrees to participate in their EHR survey, they provide survey results for free. If you are using a vendor-ranking service, make sure that they have no financial ties to vendors. In addition, medical associations, such as the American Academy of Family Physicians, often provide independent vendor surveys based on customer feedback.

9. Hold a staff meeting with those who have participated in the vendor vetting process. Gather input from key project stakeholders. Be prepared to help sell your practice on the concept of EHRs; there may be some who are not on board with this. If necessary, bring back the vendor of choice for a final validation and so that staff feels their concerns have been fully addressed. Any staff concerns should be addressed before the vendor leaves.

10. Agree on a decision to make a decision. It is important to understand that no vendor decision can be made without some unknowns and uncertainties. At this stage, the practice should make a decision to name its "vendor of choice" and begin the processes of contract negotiating. However, making a vendor-of-choice decision is not the final decision. It is simply a recognition that your practice is now ready to proceed to the final stage of the process, vendor negotiations and contracting.

REASONS FOR NOT GOING FORWARD WITH A VENDOR

This book is devoted to helping you make a good and informed vendor decision. Accordingly, we would be doing you a disservice if we did not provide you with information on how to determine when it is *not* okay to proceed with a vendor. In most cases, the "halt" order is only temporary. Nonetheless, moving forward toward contracting under any of the circumstances that follow should be avoided:

1. **Operational threats.** Although there is no "perfect" time for a practice to undergo EHR transformation, staff should not be experiencing any other major operational challenges simultaneously. For example, one should avoid EHR adoption in the middle of a merger, during leadership turnover, when undergoing facility remodeling or anything else that may distract attention from the implementation processes.

2. **Financial strains.** Every EHR transformation will add substantial financial strain to a practice's budget. A practice should never attempt an EHR transformation during difficult financial times. Although an EHR is often justified as a way to improve a practice's financial performance, the practice should be well-prepared financially for hard and soft project costs. *Hard costs* are usually predictable whereas *soft costs*—such as training expenses, lost provider productivity, and some slowdown in the revenue cycle as a result of disruptions to patient flow during project implementation—can be unknown and hard to predict. Variable expenses require that practices assume the true cost of the EHR project will be 25 to 50 percent above the vendor's proposal. According to many studies, the average cost to implement an EHR system is more than $40,000 per provider.[1]

3. **Product defects.** No matter how much you fall in love with your vendor of choice, you should never proceed with contracting when a vendor has a known product defect and they will not provide assurances that the defect will be corrected prior to system installation. Some defects can cause unwanted liabilities.

4. **Major market shift.** The EHR market is always changing and some vendors have begun discontinuing their EHRs. If, during the vendor vetting process, you discover a major change in your vendor's business status—such as mergers or acquisitions—you must put this vendor "in timeout" until you can better determine how this status change will affect your decision. You may also want to require the vendor to give you some contractual reassurance that will guarantee the ongoing viability of their software/service.

5. **Non-conforming to standards.** For your practice to qualify for ARRA financial incentives, the vendor you select will have to remain in compliance with federal and state standards. These standards are evolving continually and can change unexpectedly. In fairness, however, even vendors are unable to predict the future of compliance standards. Therefore, you should not proceed to contracting with any vendor who is unwilling to guarantee that they will keep their product/service in compliance with federal and state standards. (In Chapter 8, we provide sample contact language that will assist you in addressing this EHR contract requirement.)

CONCLUSION

EHR selection pitfalls occur when a practice fails to spend the time and effort needed up front to identify how well a vendor and their product/service aligns with the practice's known needs and expectations. Pitfalls such as allowing the vendor to rush your decision; purchasing an EHR that fails to comply with state and federal certification standards; and not building consensus within the practice are mistakes common to both EHR section and vendor vetting (as noted in Chapter 6). These pitfalls can cause a significant amount of dissatisfaction with the vendor as well as unplanned work, additional costs and even implementation failures. Every practice is unique and individual preferences will also influence the final vendor decision. Just as no EHR system is perfect, no vendor is perfect.

REFERENCE

1.   Greene J. E-records help medical groups increase savings, study finds. November 15, 2010. http://www.crainsdetroit.com/article/20101107/SUB01/311079958/e-records-help-medical-groups-increase-savings-study-finds#. Accessed December 7, 2010.

Vendor Contracting and Negotiating

INTRODUCTION

The good news for purchasers of electronic health record (EHR) solutions is that the marketplace is extremely competitive. As a result, it is a buyer's market for those willing to put forth the effort and take the time to do some deal-making. Negotiating with vendors is much more than just asking for a pricing discount, however. Deal-making should consider all aspects of the client-vendor relationship and the practice's future requirements. For example, what does the vendor charge for adding providers that may join the organization later on? How do they handle pricing increases? Does the vendor provide free upgrades, or would upgrades entail an extra expense? This chapter will help you negotiate a contract with your vendor that will protect your best interests throughout your relationship with them.

Vendors strive for success as much as you do; however, they will not volunteer to offer more favorable terms and conditions to their clients. The buyer must know what to ask for and how to go about negotiating the terms. Most vendors will consider compromises and will work with you to address your concerns regarding the contract.

NEGOTIATION BASICS

Reaching positive negotiation outcomes begins with understanding some basic principles. Here are some ground rules to help you conduct successful negotiations:

1. Never tell a vendor you are 100-percent committed to buying their system. Make sure your vendor feels like they have a creditable competitor to beat out to win your business. Establishing this leverage will help you negotiate from a position of strength.
2. Be reasonable and work to find middle ground. Negotiations are about compromising and making things fair for both parties.
3. Put together a list of what is most important and sort the list into two categories: deal breakers and wish list.
4. Avoid bad-faith negotiations. Do not commit to buy in exchange for a special requirement you do not expect to get. The vendor may "call your bluff" and agree to the requirements. Backing out can be embarrassing and uncomfortable.
5. Getting a discount is expected, but there is a fine line between getting a good deal and putting your vendor into a situation where they could lose money. You want

your vendor to be around, and you want them to feel good about helping your practice.

EHR VENDOR CONTRACT TYPES

Before getting into the major strategies for negotiating your vendor contract, first examine the types of contracts vendors offer (see Table 8-1).

Types of Vendor Contracts	Description of Contract Type
Purchase agreement	There are two forms of purchase agreement: provider license agreements and user license agreements. In both cases, the practice generally owns the software outright, but they may have to pay for future upgrades and new releases.
• Provider license agreement	The price for this form of contract is based on number of providers who use the system. Usually there is no charge for non-provider users.
• User license agreement	The price for this type of contract is based on the total number of users who have access to the system.
Concurrent user agreement	This is one of the best types of contracts in that the practice pays only for actual number of users that access the system at any given time. For example, although a practice may have 20 employees, not all of these employees will be on the system at the exact same time. A concurrent user agreement means that the price is based on system usage.
Term license	Vendors grant you a license to use the product/service for a defined period of time. These types of licenses should be avoided because repurchase is required at the end of the term.
Hosting agreement	A hosting agreement can function in the same was as any of the contracts noted above, except that the vendor hosts the software on your behalf. You still own the system, but the vendor acts as your information technology (IT) department and hosts the software from a remote data center. There is generally an extra monthly fee for this service.
Application service provider (ASP)	A true ASP is a vendor that provides the software to you via the Internet for a monthly subscription fee. This contract option is often confused with hosting agreements, which, as noted above, is when your system being hosted off-site. With an ASP, you never own the system; instead, you subscribe to it.

Table 8-1: Types of Contracts Offered by Vendors

Types of Vendor Contracts	Description of Contract Type
Software as a service (SaaS)	This arrangement is very similar to an ASP. However, SaaS is 100 percent Web based and would never run on-premises. SaaS is the current trend because there are usually no up-front costs and it is 100 percent turnkey. The system is always current with this system/contract type; all updates and enhancements are provided at no additional charge.
Free software	Believe it or not, there are free EHRs on the market. Generally, a trade-off is involved, such as being exposed to advertising or research. These systems are usually financially backed by companies who want clinical data that should be protected in accordance with current state and federal regulations.

Table 8-1: *(Continued)*

Reading the Fine Print

Understanding the details of negotiating and contracting with vendors requires that you read all of the document's fine print.

A vendor's standard software license or subscription agreement is filled with vendor-favorable terms and conditions, containing provisions that serve and protect only the vendor. License limitations, disclaimers, exceptions, licensee duties and prohibitions, vendor rights, and so on, are all to the benefit of the vendor. In fact, very little in a standard contract protects the purchaser or subscriber. To modify a contract to serve and protect the buyer calls for knowing what to ask for and how to negotiate for it. As a result, this chapter is dedicated to bringing some transparency to the process. It provides some practical tips on how to negotiate a vendor contact.

Knowledge is power—and the key to success. However, this chapter should not be considered legal advice and it does not take the place of legal counsel. It is also impossible to cover or address every scenario or situation that might arise in the purchase of EHR solutions. Table 8-2 suggests some of the major areas you may wish to address in your vendor contract.

As previously stated, the sample contract language provided in this chapter should not be considered legal advice, nor should this chapter take the place of consulting with an attorney or expert in vendor contracting.

Contract Requirement	Definition and Sample Contract Language
Entity relation-ship diagrams (ERDs) upon request	An ERD allows a customer to see how the vendor's database is configured. This information is helpful when your IT staff attempts to develop interfaces and create special reports. Obtaining this diagram in advance will also prevent unexpected fees later, should you determine that you need this information after the contract is signed. ***SAMPLE CONTRACT LANGUAGE:*** *The Company will supply Customer with entity relationship diagrams (ERDs) upon request in order to permit Customer to analyze database structure so that the data can be stored and retrieved in a most efficient manner.*
Acceptance period	An acceptance period is one of the most important requirements for vendor contracting. The acceptance period states that although you agree to enter into a contract, you do not accept the contract as final until certain conditions are satisfied and confirmed. ***SAMPLE CONTRACT LANGUAGE:*** *Software Acceptance. Customer will accept the Software and System ninety (90) days after the successful installation, implementation, and use of each module pertaining to the Software and System. Software not properly installed or Software installation not completed by the Company (including System third-party software), will be corrected at the Company's expense, including travel expenses for on-site work.* *The parties will agree upon an "Acceptance Plan" as part of the Software installation and any "Programs." The Acceptance Plan will include implementation team training for Customer personnel and for the purpose of verifying and confirming performance in accordance to the Documentation and specifications of the Software. Company represents and warrants that the media and other information provided by Company for the Software installation will include, among other items and information, sample data designed to assist in testing and verification that the System is successfully installed and performing specified procedures meeting all published specifications for the current version of the Programs.* *The Acceptance Plan will include at a minimum five (5) levels of review as stated below:* *1. Level 1 Software reviews to ensure that the information, screen, and data flows represent those shown in the Documentation.* *2. Level 2 Software reviews to determine that data elements within the applications are consistent with the Documentation.* *3. Level 3 Software reviews to determine all edits, calculations, and logic are consistent with the Documentation.*

Table 8-2: Contract Requirements

Contract Requirement	Definition and Sample Contract Language
Acceptance period *(continued)*	4. *Level 4 Software reviews to determine that all reports, both online and batch, daily, and periodic, are consistent with the Documentation. In addition, all data transfer or interfaces within the scope of this Agreement, the Addendum, and all Appendices are functioning per specification.* 5. *Level 5 Software reviews to determine that performance of primary documented operations procedures produce the results described in the Documentation.*
Implementation	Implementation makes or breaks the EHR project. You should expect only the most qualified vendor staff working on your project. **SAMPLE CONTRACT LANGUAGE:** *All personnel serving on the implementation team/trainers must have a minimum of two (2) years employment with the Company in their current role. The Customer does not agree to accept and will not be obligated to accept any Company trainers or other Company personnel providing service hereunder with less than two (2) years of implementation experience. The Customer may also request and Company will provide from time to time substitute staff if required by Customer.*
Support fees	Most vendors will try to start charging monthly support fees as soon as the contract is signed. You should never start paying for support until the system is successfully installed to your satisfaction and you can verify that requirements from the acceptance period have been accomplished. **SAMPLE CONTRACT LANGUAGE:** *Support will be charged applicable to what is installed. Customer's obligation to make support fee payments will commence ninety (90) days after the successful installation, implementation, and use of the Software and System. If the practice is installing multiple modules, Company will only charge Customer support for the portion installed commencing ninety (90) days after the successful installation, implementation, and use of each such module pertaining to the Software and System.*

Table 8-2: *(Continued)*

Contract Requirement	Definition and Sample Contract Language

Assignment	**Important:** Software is nontransferable! This lack of transferability is a potential problem for most medical practices because the practice may eventually be sold or acquired by another owner. It is very important to make sure your vendor allows you to transfer your software contract under any circumstance.
	
	SAMPLE CONTRACT LANGUAGE:
	Notwithstanding any other term of condition in the Agreement, Company will allow and hereby consents to assignment of the Software and System under any of the following conditions or to any of the following organizations:
	  • *merger – to the successor,*
	  • *acquisition – to the buyer,*
	  • *buy-out,*
	  • *name change,*
	  • *corporate reorganization,*
	  • *successor organization,*
	  • *parent organization,*
	  • *subsidiary or affiliate,*
	  • *or to another entity within the same organization as Customer.*

Relocation	Some vendor contracts prohibit relocating the system without first getting the vendor's approval or paying the vendor for relocation services. Most vendors will not prevent you from relocating the system, but it is best to reach an understanding in advance to avoid any extra charges. *SAMPLE CONTRACT LANGUAGE:* *Customer may, at its sole discretion upon notice to Company, relocate its servers or other Hardware. The Company will provide support for this relocation under the maintenance agreement or at the published hourly rates.*

Table 8-2: *(Continued)*

Contract Requirement	Definition and Sample Contract Language
Future upgrades	**Deal Breaker!** Never buy any system without an agreement obligating the vendor to provide future system upgrades. Unexpected state and federal mandates can happen without notice. The vendor must conform to these requirements and make sure their system stays modern and current. Vendors have been known to sell a version of software, and then later discontinue it, requiring their customers to purchase an upgraded version. This practice should not be allowed because it is a certainty that vendors will have to provide future upgrades to stay in compliance with government mandates including EHR certification requirements. *SAMPLE CONTRACT LANGUAGE:* *The Company will provide to Customer continuous and unlimited use and right to under this Agreement and Addendum upgrades, new releases, version changes, mandated modifications and patches to the Software and System under the Service Agreement, the Agreement, and this Addendum at no additional cost. Training and installation to support new releases, upgrades, and patches will be covered under the standard maintenance agreement. The Company will provide continued support for previous versions of its Software for a period of ten (10) years. Additionally, the Customer will not be charged for any mandatory Software modification to meet any and all compliance requirements (federal, state, or local).*
Government mandates and certification	**Deal Breaker!** Vendors are expected to meet federal compliance standards on a myriad of levels. It is not possible to define these standards herein because they are always evolving. A vendor who is committed to staying in the market will make a commitment to meet and conform to these standards. *SAMPLE CONTRACT LANGUAGE:* *The Company will comply with all government mandates and standards and will modify the Software accordingly at no additional cost to Customer.*

Table 8-2: *(Continued)*

Contract Requirement	Definition and Sample Contract Language
Third-party software	Most vendors rely on third-party software to run their applications. For example, most vendors recommend a specific operating system or database, such as Microsoft SQL or Oracle. The vendor must be responsible for how their software performs on these third-party components and must provide the necessary troubleshooting to solve any issues that arise. **SAMPLE CONTRACT LANGUAGE:** *The Customer expects third-party software recommended by the Company to perform as required and to be compatible with the Software or System. The Customer will use commercially reasonable efforts to purchase the recommended third-party software in accordance to the Company's requirements. The Company will pay the replacement cost or cost to purchase alternative third-party software if the recommended third-party software does not meet the requirements or if it compromises the performance of the Software or System.*
Copyright infringement	Although rare, a vendor could violate a copyright infringement and be forced to discontinue selling their software or the portion that violates the copyright infringement. Should this happen, the vendor must refund or provide an alternative solution to its customers. **SAMPLE CONTRACT LANGUAGE:** *Company represents and warrants to Customer that it has full right, title, and interest in and to the Software. Furthermore, Company agrees to indemnify and hold harmless the Customer, its affiliates, and assignees from and against any claim, suit, or liability arising out of or related to copyright infringement claims against the Software. Company agrees to indemnify and protect Customer from any and all expenses or costs, including attorneys' fees, hardware, and professional expenses (including travel) if the Software is in violation of copyright infringements. Notwithstanding any other term or condition in the Agreement or this Addendum, nothing herein will obligate Customer to accept or utilize any alternative software in the event of or as the result of any litigation, court decree or order, or settlement agreement related to the Software. Company, in the event Customer is no longer permitted to use the Software as the result of any litigation, court decree or order, or settlement agreement related to the Software, will pay to Customer a business-disruption fee equal to twenty-five percent (25%) of the Customer's annual net revenue arising out of or related to the practices of its employed physicians. Such payment is in the form of liquidated damages and not a penalty, and will be due within ten (10) business days of demand by Customer. The parties agree that a calculation of damages in such event would be difficult and that such amount is reasonable under the circumstances.*

Table 8-2: *(Continued)*

Contract Requirement	Definition and Sample Contract Language
Warranties	**Deal Breaker!** It is critical to thoroughly review and understand the warranty provided by the vendor. Most vendor warranties last for only 90 days, and almost all such terms start at contract signing. In some cases, therefore, the warranty will expire before the software is installed. A warranty should start after the software goes live and meets the requirements of the acceptance period. *SAMPLE CONTRACT LANGUAGE:* *Company guarantees, represents, and warrants to Customer that Company will correct or repair any errors, malfunctions, or performance defects or provide a reasonable substitution to the Software within ninety (90) days ("Error Correction Period") after Company reports such errors, malfunctions, or performance defects to Company ("Error Notification Date"). If Company is not able to correct or repair such errors, malfunctions, or performance defects in the Software within the Error Correction Period or cannot correct or install a reasonable substitution within the Error Correction Period, Company will pay and refund to Customer all expenses paid to the Company, including Hardware and expenses paid for professional services, including travel expenses.*
Interfaces	All vendors offer and provide interfacing. Interfacing is always a two-party dance between vendors. Conflicts are common and one vendor may even try to sabotage the other as a way of discouraging the interfacing of competing products. Most interfaces can be verified before contracting; however, your contract must hold the vendor accountable and responsible for ensuring the interface stays in working order after the sale. *SAMPLE CONTRACT LANGUAGE:* *Notwithstanding any provision of Section 7 or elsewhere in the Agreement, the Company represents and warrants to Customer that Company will for each Interface purchased by Customer perform, support, and troubleshoot Interfaces as a part of the annual maintenance agreement. Company will support modifications and version changes to Interfaces at no additional cost to Company. Company will provide any Interface already written at no additional cost to Customer. Company will refund the cost of the Interface if it becomes nonfunctional and is not corrected within ninety (90) days by Company after notice by Customer.*

Table 8-2: *(Continued)*

Contract Requirement	Definition and Sample Contract Language
Confidentiality	Most vendor contracts prohibit customers from seeking outside assistance to solve technical problems. Some vendor contracts even try to prevent customers from making negative statements about their products. You must always reserve the right to seek help from someone other than your vendor without any violation to your contract or warranty. *SAMPLE CONTRACT LANGUAGE:* *Company will allow the Customer to provide outside consultants or legal counsel access to Confidential Information. The Customer will request that any third party execute a nondisclosure agreement before releasing any Confidential Information. Notwithstanding any other term or condition of the Agreement, any Appendices or attachments or this Addendum, Confidential Information will not include information that (i) was in the possession of either party before its disclosure by the disclosing party; (ii) is disclosed to either party by an independent source having no legal obligation of confidentiality to the disclosing party; and/or (iii) is or becomes generally available to the public or to persons in the healthcare industry other than through a breach of this Agreement.*
Effects of termination	Terminating a vendor contract is not something you plan for when buying a system. However, having an exit strategy is critical and can save you a lot of heartache and headaches in the future should you have to cross that bridge. Some vendor contracts require their customers to discontinue use of the system and to destroy the software. Others prohibit data conversions and/or system access after termination. A vendor can also impose whatever fees they want and will usually find ways to make it expensive to terminate their services. *SAMPLE CONTRACT LANGUAGE:* *Upon termination, Company will provide to Customer de-conversion file in an American Standard Code for Information Interchange (ASCII) and/or RTF (rich text format) or other document file format acceptable to Customer that is capable of storing documents on a storage media. The Company will agree to provide one test tape and one live data tape in the format noted above. At no time will the Company terminate or shut down the Software without the Customer's prior approval. Customer will be allowed an indefinite amount of time to transition off of the Software. Company will provide any reasonable and necessary support to Customer to facilitate any transition at the published hourly rate of Company and Company will cooperate with any new or replacement vendor selected by Customer to coordinate the transition.*

Table 8-2: *(Continued)*

Contract Requirement	Definition and Sample Contract Language
Effects of termination (continued)	*Customer may terminate the Agreement, the Appendices, and this Addendum for any reason upon provision of ninety (90) days notice to Company. If either party terminates the Agreement prior to the expiration of the term, for any reason, unless provided for elsewhere, Customer will only be responsible for payments due up until the date of termination. Any prepaid amounts made by Customer that are not actually due until after the date of termination will be refunded to Customer within five (5) business days of the date of termination of the Agreement. In the event Customer or Hospital, alone or as a member of a healthcare system, elects to merge, discontinue, downsize, integrate, restructure, or otherwise materially alter the services to be performed hereunder, Customer will provide Company with at least sixty (60) days notice prior to a termination under this Section.*
Malware or Trojan horses	Some vendors will install disabling software that will allow them to shut off your system remotely in the event of a contract dispute. A vendor should never be allowed to shut off your system under any circumstances. They can refuse to provide support, but shutting off the system should be strictly prohibited. ***SAMPLE CONTRACT LANGUAGE:*** *Under no circumstances can Company disable or shut off Customer's System.*
Default	This describes what happens should the vendor default on any portion of your contract. ***SAMPLE CONTRACT LANGUAGE:*** *In the event Company defaults in the performance of any terms of this Agreement, delivers to Customer Software that does not conform to written acceptance criteria as defined in the Agreement or this Addendum, or otherwise breaches the Agreement or this Addendum and Company fails to take action to correct such default or breach within a reasonable period of time after written notice has been given by Customer, or such longer period not to exceed thirty (30) days as may be required so long as Company is proceeding diligently, Customer may terminate this Agreement and Customer will not be obligated to make any additional payments to Company. In the event that Customer elects to terminate this Agreement due to the failure of Company to remedy its breach of this Agreement, Customer will have the right to retain and use the Software indefinitely from the date of termination to permit Customer's migration to a suitable replacement system. Customer will pay Company's support and maintenance fees for the period of use at the published rate.*

Table 8-2: *(Continued)*

Contract Requirement	Definition and Sample Contract Language
Source code	**Deal Breaker!** The source code is necessary to reverse engineer your system and remove your data in the event your vendor goes out of business or discontinues their software without offering an alternative. Most vendors will agree to enroll your practice with a source code agent who will provide the source code to all the vendor's customers should there be a qualifying event. *SAMPLE CONTRACT LANGUAGE:* *Company will agree to secure the source code or the Software in an escrow account to be released to the Company in the event of bankruptcy, liquidation, or sale and will release all manuals, passwords, and any other security information about the Software. Company will pay the Customer's cost of setting up the escrow account to hold the source code. If the Company has a national escrow account, Company will provide to Customer upon the execution of the Agreement, and annually thereafter, proof of registration.*
Future providers/users	Now is the time to understand how the vendor will charge the practice to add providers to the EHR system in the future. Once you sign the contract, you will no longer have any leverage to secure discounts. This is the best time to have your vendor agree to future pricing. *SAMPLE CONTRACT LANGUAGE:* *Company acknowledges that Customer will experience economies of scale when adding future users/providers and agrees to allow Customer to have future provider/users added at the same percentage of discount based on current day published pricing.* *Increases to Support Fees. The Company can increase its support fees only at the rate of one percent (1%) less than the consumer price index. In addition, the Company cannot look back for more than a one (1) year period if the fee is not increased.*
Unforeseen support	Unforeseen circumstances are common but generally unavoidable. Vendors should be required to obtain your approval and authorization before invoicing the practice to address unforeseen issues. *SAMPLE CONTRACT LANGUAGE:* *Unforeseen requests, customizations, and other services outside of the scope of this Agreement will be mutually agreed to. Company agrees to provide additional service at the discounted rate. Company also warrants deliverables by correcting issues as agreed and correcting any subsequent issues resulting from these modifications.* *Decrease Number in Providers. If the Customer reduces its number of providers, the Company will reduce its maintenance costs as applicable.*

Table 8-2: *(Continued)*

Contract Requirement	Definition and Sample Contract Language
Discontinuation of support	Your practice may reach a point of fluency with the EHR system that the annual technical support subscription no longer seems necessary. If your practice rarely uses technical support services, it may be more economical to pay for this service based on actual usage. We offer one word of caution, however; maintenance fees should never be discontinued because that service allows you to receive ongoing upgrades and enhancements. Most vendors are able to unbundle maintenance and support to allow their customers to drop support when it is no longer needed. *SAMPLE CONTRACT LANGUAGE:* *Customer may elect to discontinue maintenance upon provision of ninety (90) days notice to Company. If support is required after terminating the maintenance contract, Company will charge its published hourly rate for support on an as-needed basis and its applicable rate for any additional releases or upgrades.*
Good customer discount	Vendors will often give their long-term customers a "good customer discount" when support utilization drops. This discount would be in lieu of discontinuing support. *SAMPLE CONTRACT LANGUAGE:* *Company acknowledges and agrees that the Customer will become more efficient with the Software over time. In accordance, the Company will agree to give the Customer a good customer discount, or forty percent (40%) of the annual support cost, if support utilization becomes minimal.*
Additional training	Vendors frequently provide routine training in classrooms or via the Internet. These training courses are not exclusive to any one customer. Vendors should be willing to allow your practice to participate in community training programs at no additional cost. *SAMPLE CONTRACT LANGUAGE:* *Reinforcement Training/Ongoing Training. Customer will have the opportunity to continue Software/System education by attending the following Company resource education sessions at no additional charge: user conference, Internet-based training, and classroom training at the Company's office. Additional training performed at the Customer's site will be at the Company's applicable rates. Company also agrees to provide reinforcement training after go-live at no cost if the initial training does not meet the requirements of the Customer.*

Table 8-2: *(Continued)*

Contract Requirement	Definition and Sample Contract Language
Non-covered services	Services not included in the standard contract require approval in advance of providing the service. **SAMPLE CONTRACT LANGUAGE:** *During the term hereof, Company and Customer will mutually agree on non-covered services. Customer agrees to pay to Company the same discounted hourly rate for any services outside of this Agreement. Company provides this provision in lieu of offering a "guarantee not to exceed." Customer understands that not all services are capable of being defined at the execution of the Agreement and this Addendum.*
Showroom site	Vendors frequently offer their customers the opportunity to become a showroom site. Showroom sites are usually responsible for hosting site visits for potential EHR buyers and demonstrating best practices on how to use the software. It is customary for the vendor to compensate the practice that takes on the role of showroom site. **SAMPLE CONTRACT LANGUAGE:** *Showroom Site/Site Visits. Company may request from time to time to use the Customer's physician practice as a reference site. Company must request permission and the Customer reserves the right to decline the request for any reason or no reason. Company will issue a support credit of one thousand and 00/100 dollars ($1,000.00) for each hosted visit. Company will be required to have its guests sign confidentially statements and/or Business Associate Agreements or other privacy agreements before arriving at one or more of the Company's practice sites. Company will pay to Customer an agreed upon fee of five percent (5%) of the sale if the site visit results in a purchase.*
Documentation	Most vendors provide their policies and training manuals online. It is also a good policy to have the vendor provide your practice with a hard copy of all documents and manuals for safekeeping. **SAMPLE CONTRACT LANGUAGE:** *Company will provide the Customer with any and all Documentation and will continue to provide Documentation updates during the course of the relationship. Company will not charge the Customer for this Documentation. Company will make available to the Customer and will make reasonable efforts to assist the Customer with using this information and knowledge.*
Data mining	Vendors should be restricted from mining or accessing your practice's data without prior approval. **SAMPLE CONTRACT LANGUAGE:** *Clinical Content and Data Mining. Customer does not allow any access to its clinical content and does not authorize the Company to conduct any data mining without authorization.*

Table 8-2: *(Continued)*

Contract Requirement	Definition and Sample Contract Language
Electronic data interchange (EDI) services	Most vendors required the use of an EDI vendor to help with transmitting claims and for remittance. Your vendor should be responsible for providing support between their software and the EDI vendor. *SAMPLE CONTRACT LANGUAGE:* *Company will support electronic data interchange (EDI) functions and will work with the clearinghouse to resolve issues. EDI services must be functional and working properly before final payment.*
Solicitation	Vendors frequently hire their staff away from their customers. This form of recruiting should be discouraged to prevent practice turnover. *SAMPLE CONTRACT LANGUAGE:* *Solicitation. Company will not make any attempt to solicit employees from the Customer without obtaining permission.*
Emergency support	Most vendors have a support policy that reflects different levels of responsiveness based on problem urgency. Emergency support should be a contractual obligation. *SAMPLE CONTRACT LANGUAGE:* *Company will provide twenty-four (24)-hour emergency support seven (7) days a week 365 days per year during the term hereof. Company agrees to the following response time: one (1) hour for urgent/critical calls (this may need to be defined), eight (8) hours for non-urgent/critical calls, twenty-four (24) hours for general questions.*
Travel policy	Vendors will typically have an enforceable travel policy required for their staff. Be sure to inspect the travel policy to ensure there are some limitations. Vendors should be required to get prior approval before booking any airline ticket that costs more than $500.00. Daily expenses should be capped on a per diem basis. *SAMPLE CONTRACT LANGUAGE:* *Travel Policy. The Company will agree to a travel policy.*
Access	With the exception of routine support, vendors should provide advance notice before accessing your system. *SAMPLE CONTRACT LANGUAGE:* *The Company must seek prior approval from Customer before accessing the Customer's server or workstations.*
Audit	From time to time, a vendor may conduct an audit to ensure their system is being used in accordance to their policies. The vendor should be required to provide prior notice and state the reason for the audit. *SAMPLE CONTRACT LANGUAGE:* *Company must notify the Customer sixty (60) days prior to an audit by Company. Company must state the reason for the audit and provide written explanation of the outcome. All confidentiality provisions will apply to any such audit.*

Table 8-2: *(Continued)*

Contract Requirement	Definition and Sample Contract Language
Payment terms	**Deal Breaker!** Vendors will generally require their customers to pay 50 percent on contract signing and 50 percent thirty (30) days after they ship the software. This arrangement is unacceptable. The vendor should base their payment terms on deliverables and accomplishments. Using a time line based on dates does not ensure the system is working before a payment is expected. Payments should be based on project milestones. Here is an easy example of a reasonable payment term policy. *SAMPLE CONTRACT LANGUAGE:* *Payment Terms and Conditions.* *Twenty-five percent (25%) at signing of this Agreement.* *Twenty-five percent (25%) after successful loading of Software.* *Twenty-five percent (25%) after successful training.* *Twenty-five percent (25%) after successful go-live.* *Annual support starts sixty (60) days after go-live.* *Professional services paid as incurred.* *Travel expenses paid as incurred.*
Corporate compliance	Policies vary by company, but you should always include any corporate compliance policies necessary for suppliers to follow. *SAMPLE CONTRACT LANGUAGE:* *Corporate Compliance. Customer has developed and implemented a Corporate Compliance Plan to ensure all business activity is conducted in accordance with all federal, state, and other laws and regulations as appropriate. Company hereby agrees that it will comply with Customer's Corporate Compliance Plan and will conduct its business in accordance with all federal, state, and other laws and regulations as appropriate. The parties warrant that they are in good standing with all federal and state programs, and that they are properly qualified, licensed, registered, and/or certified in conformity with federal and state laws and regulations. Should either party's status in regard to same change, that party will notify the other party immediately, and the party that is notified will have the right to immediately terminate this Agreement. The parties agree to not knowingly participate in any activity pursuant to this Agreement or in any aspect of the relationship that may constitute or be construed to constitute a violation of federal or state laws or regulations, including but not limited to improper arrangements or referrals under the Ethics in Patient Referral Act, Title 42 of the United States Code Section 1395nn (a.k.a. the Stark law), the federal anti-kickback statute, Title 42 of the United States Code Section 1320a-7b(b), or the Health Insurance Portability and Accountability Act, 104 P.L. 191, 110 Stat. 1936 (1996). The parties agree to take all reasonable precautions to avoid the same.*

Table 8-2: *(Continued)*

Contract Requirement	Definition and Sample Contract Language
Indemnification	**Deal Breaker!** If the vendor's software malfunctions and creates an unwanted liability, the vendor must step in and defend the practice and physician/user. *SAMPLE CONTRACT LANGUAGE:* *Indemnification. Each party agrees to indemnify and hold the other party, and its respective directors and officers, forever harmless from and against any and all liabilities, demands, claims, actions, or causes of action, assessments, judgments, losses, costs, damages, or expenses, including reasonable attorneys' fees, sustained or incurred by the other party resulting from or arising out of or by virtue of: the discharge of its obligations under this Agreement; noncompliance with or breach by such party or any of its employees or agents of any of the covenants, commitments, or obligations of this Agreement to be performed by such party; or any negligent or willful act or omission by such party or its employees, directors, officers, or agents, which acts or omissions result in any bodily injury.*
Notice	Each party should agree to provide proper notice before taking any action. *SAMPLE CONTRACT LANGUAGE:* *Notice. In the event that any claim is asserted against a party that is entitled to indemnification hereunder, such party ("indemnified party") will promptly after learning of such claim notify the party obligated to indemnify it ("indemnifying party") thereof in writing. The failure of the indemnified party, however, to give prompt notice of such claim will not relieve the obligation of the indemnifying party with respect to such claim. Except to the extent otherwise provided by the terms of applicable insurance policies (other than self-insurance), the indemnifying party will have the right, upon written notice to the indemnified party within ten (10) business days after receipt from the indemnified party of notice of such claim, to conduct at its expense the defense against such claim in its own name, or, if the indemnifying party will fail to give such notice, it will be deemed to have elected not to conduct the defense of the subject claim and, in such event, the indemnified party will have the right to conduct such defense and to compromise and settle the claim without prior consent of the indemnifying party. In the event that the indemnifying party elects to conduct the defense of the subject claim, the indemnified party will cooperate with and make available to the indemnifying party such assistance and materials as may be reasonably requested, all at the expense of the indemnifying party. The indemnified party will have the right, at its expense, to participate in the defense, provided that the indemnified party will have the right to compromise and settle the claim only with the prior written consent of the indemnifying party, unless otherwise provided by the terms of applicable insurance policies.*

Table 8-2: *(Continued)*

Contract Requirement	Definition and Sample Contract Language
Outside contractors	This clause establishes the vendor as an independent contractor so it is clear that they are responsible for all their own obligations under employment law and to the Internal Revenue Service. *SAMPLE CONTRACT LANGUAGE:* *Independent Contractor. The parties agree that they are independent businesses and function as independent contractors in relation to each other. On this basis, the parties have and will maintain sole financial responsibility for payment of all of their own taxes, unemployment, workers' compensation, and other such withholding or insurance on account of their own performances under the terms of this Agreement as independent contractors.*
Governing law	**Deal Breaker!** Every vendor contract states that the law governing the relationship is to be that of the state of the vendor. Should an issue arise requiring legal action, you would be required to travel to the vendor's state to take legal action. Most vendors will agree to move governing law to the state of their customer. A reasonable compromise would be to select a state other than that where the vendor or practice is located to make it mutually inconvenient to go to court. We strongly recommend moving governing law to the state where the software will be used. *SAMPLE CONTRACT LANGUAGE:* *Interpretation, Jurisdiction, and Venue. This Agreement will be deemed to have been made in the state/commonwealth of (YOUR STATE) and will be governed by and construed in accordance with (YOUR STATE) law. The parties agree to submit any and all disputes arising out of this Agreement, including its interpretation, exclusively to the state/commonwealth or federal courts of (YOUR STATE).*
Severability	This clause ensures that your contract terms remain in effect even if ownership of the vendor changes. *SAMPLE CONTRACT LANGUAGE:* *Severability. The provisions of this Agreement are intended to be severable and enforced to the maximum extent permitted by law. If for any reason any provision of this Agreement will be held to be invalid, illegal, or unenforceable in whole or in part in any jurisdiction, then that provision will be ineffective only to the extent of the determined invalidity, illegality, or unenforceability, and in that jurisdiction only, without in any manner affecting the validity, legality, or enforceability of the unaffected portion, and the other provisions in that jurisdiction or any provision of the Agreement in any other jurisdiction. The unaffected portion and provisions of the Agreement will be enforced to the maximum extent permitted by law.*

Table 8-2: *(Continued)*

Contract Requirement	Definition and Sample Contract Language
Access to records	Should there be an audit of any kind or investigation for a software malfunction that created a liability, your practice must have the rights to access the vendor's records and their documentation.
	SAMPLE CONTRACT LANGUAGE:
	Access to Books, Documents, and Records. Company will provide Customer and its representatives access to the database for any adult patient for a period of seven (7) years from the date of termination of this Agreement and seventeen (17) years from the date of termination of the Agreement and this Addendum for any newborn or pediatric patient.
	For a period of four (4) years after the expiration or termination of this Agreement, Company will make available, upon request from the Secretary of Health and Human Services, the Comptroller General of the United States, or any of their duly authorized representatives, this Agreement and books, documents, and records of the Company that are necessary to verify the nature and extent of the costs of the services provided hereunder by Company, in accordance with applicable U.S. government regulations in effect from time to time. If Company carries out any of its duties under this Agreement through a subcontract with a related organization, the value or cost of which is $10,000.00 or more during a twelve (12) month period, such subcontract will contain a clause to the effect that until the expiration of four (4) years after the furnishing of services pursuant to such subcontract, the related organization will make available, upon request from Secretary of Health and Human Services, the Comptroller General of the United States, or any of their duly authorized representatives, the subcontract and books, documents, and records of the related organization that are necessary to verify the nature and extent of such costs.

Table 8-2: *(Continued)*

Contract Requirement	Definition and Sample Contract Language
Sanction provider	This eventuality is unlikely, but it requires the vendor to confirm they are not under any investigation or audit under Medicare or Medicaid, nor have they been restricted as a sanctioned provider. *SAMPLE CONTRACT LANGUAGE:* *Company represents and warrants that neither it nor its employees, contractors, or agents are or have ever been a "Sanctioned Provider." For purposes of this Agreement, a "Sanctioned Provider" means a Person who is currently under indictment or prosecution for, or has been convicted of: (i) any offense related to the delivery of an item or service under the Medicare or Medicaid programs or any program funded under Title V or Title XX of the Social Security Act (the Maternal and Child Health Services Program or the Block Grants to States for Social Services programs, respectively), (ii) a criminal offense relating to neglect or abuse of patients in connection with the delivery of a healthcare item or service, (iii) fraud, theft, embezzlement, or other financial misconduct in connection with the delivery of a health-care item or service, (iv) obstructing an investigation of any crime referred to in items (i) through (iii), above, or (v) unlawful manufacture, distribution, prescription, or dispensing of a controlled substance; has been required to pay any civil monetary penalty under 42 U.S.C. § 1320a-7a regarding false, fraudulent, or impermissible claims under, or payments to induce a reduction or limitation of healthcare services to beneficiaries of, any state or federal healthcare program, or is currently the subject of any investigation or proceeding which may result in such payment; or has been excluded from participation in the Medicare, Medicaid, or Maternal and Child Health Services (Title V) program, or any program funded under the Block Grants to States for Social Services (Title XX) program.*

Table 8-2: *(Continued)*

Contract Requirement	Definition and Sample Contract Language
Health Insurance Portability and Accountability Act of 1996 (HIPAA)	In addition to standard business associates agreements, your vendor should be contractually required to conform to all HIPAA policies and mandates. *SAMPLE CONTRACT LANGUAGE:* *HIPAA. Company agrees to abide by Sections 261 through 264 of the federal Health Insurance Portability and Accountability Act of 1996, Public Law 104-191, known as "the Administrative Simplification provisions" and any and all standards to protect the security, confidentiality, and integrity of health information promulgated by the Department of Health and Human Services and Company in the treatment of any patient information obtained or derived from Customer or any affiliate (the "HIPAA Privacy and Security Rules"). In the event of an inconsistency between the provisions of this Agreement and Addendum and mandatory provisions of the HIPAA Privacy and Security Rules, as amended, the HIPAA Privacy and Security Rules in effect at the time will control. The provisions of this Agreement are intended to establish the minimum requirements regarding Company's use and disclosure of protected health information. Company agrees to use and implement appropriate administrative, physical, and technical safeguards that reasonably and appropriately protect the confidentiality, integrity, and availability of the protected health information that it creates, receives, maintains, or transmits on behalf of the Company and to prevent use or disclosure of such information other than as provided for by this Agreement.*

Table 8-2: *(Continued)*

Contract Requirement	Definition and Sample Contract Language
Stimulus incentives	**Deal Breaker!** Vendor must agree to conform to all current and future stimulus compliance mandates. Software providers must develop their programs to conform to certain functionality standards. These standards will evolve over time; therefore, the vendor must agree to conform to standards that are currently unknown. *SAMPLE CONTRACT LANGUAGE:* *a. All versions of the Software necessary to satisfy all requirements in order to be a Certified EHR (as defined below) for use by Customer to receive all of the Medicare incentives available under The Health Information Technology for Economic and Clinical Health Act (HITECH) beginning on October 1, 2010, and will not be subject to any reduction in reimbursement as a result of Customer failure to use a "certified EHR" as a "meaningful user." Such Software shall be provided (1) with respect to the initial definition of Certified EHR, at least _____ months prior to October 1, 2010, and (2) if the definition of Certified EHR is revised thereafter, an updated version of the Software that satisfies each such revised definition at least ____ months before the revised definition of Certified EHR becomes effective. Such new versions may be referred to as "Certified EHR Versions."* *As used herein, the terms "Certified EHR" and "meaningful user" each has the respective meanings assigned to such terms in HITECH (and any subsequent amendments thereto) and in the regulations promulgated from time to time pursuant to HITECH, including the most recent versions of HITECH and such regulations. All implementation, training, data conversion, and other services that may be necessary or appropriate to reasonably assist Customer in implementing each of the Certified EHR Versions that Customer may, in its discretion, elect to implement by way of becoming a "meaningful user."*
Unique requirements	Add any contractual terms that you believe are necessary for your practice to achieve a successful installation or adoption.
Vendor promises	During the sales process, the vendor may have made several promises, such as a time line for completing the installation or an offer of extra services. As it is always advisable to get these types of promises in writing, add them to the terms of your contract.

Table 8-2: *(Continued)*

Contract Requirement	Definition and Sample Contract Language
The request for proposal (RFP) tool	If you used an RFP, make sure the contract is tied back to it. ***SAMPLE CONTRACT LANGUAGE:*** *By signing below, the agent or representative of the Company does so with the express intent of certifying that all information that has been set forth in this request for proposal is accurate and in line with that which the Company can provide.* *Furthermore, by signing this document, the agent/representative of the Company acknowledges that any of the information set forth can potentially be requested to be a part or accompany the particular System that is selected. Although we acknowledge that certain issues may arise when implementing a System of this size, we agree not to hold the Company responsible for such issues that we consider unavoidable or undisclosed in this RFP dated _____.* *However, if it appears that any agent/representative of the Company has provided information that is untrue, or if it becomes evident that there are products or services that the Company's agent/representative has assured the Customer they would receive but are not in existence or if there will be an additional, nominal charge above that which was estimated, the Company reserves the right to terminate any and all discussions, negotiations, and/or implementation processes that have been conducted with the Company up to that point.* *The Company agent/representative signing this Agreement agrees that he/she is in a position within the Company that allows them to make commitments similar to those that have been set forth in this Agreement. If it is determined at a later date that this agent/representative was not in a position to make such commitments, the Customer reserves the right to terminate all discussions, negotiations, and/or implementations that have been made with the Company up to that point.*

Table 8-2: *(Continued)*

PRICE NEGOTIATIONS

The final section of this chapter covers negotiating the EHR system pricing. Typically vendor discounts can range from 5 to 50 percent of the published price and varies based on the number of providers and the amount of software that is a part of the contract. In every deal, there are usually seven "buckets" of cost that warrant attention. Here is a list of each bucket and some tips for negotiating the price of each.

1. **Software costs.** This cost is typically based on the number of users. Vendors have the most flexibility for discounting on software because it is a nontangible item. It also does not cost the vendor any extra overhead to sell one license or ten licenses. Thus, discounting on software should be the one area where the vendor has the most pricing flexibility.

2. **Professional services costs.** Typically, this cost is based on the vendor's estimates for the number of staff hours they will need to install the entire system. Currently, the industry average for professional services ranges from $100.00 to $250.00 an hour, depending on the type of experts being used. Most vendors will agree to give some discounts on their professional services. However, the vendor does in fact incur a hard cost for staff time, so you should expect that discounting for professional services will be relatively low compared with that available for software.

3. **Hardware costs.** This cost is typically driven based on pre-defined specifications and will generally come from third-party suppliers. Hardware is hardware and costs are usually dictated by the manufacturing process. Some vendors have secured special pricing by working directly with manufacturers and will allow savings to be passed on to their clients. Other vendors take the opposite approach and mark up the hardware and resell it. An easy way to find out if you are getting a good deal on your hardware is to conduct a fast Internet search for pricing options. On average, vendors should have a 5 to 10 percent margin on hardware to offer to their clients.

4. **Maintenance and support costs.** Software support typically ranges from 18 to 25 percent of the cost of the software. Keeping down maintenance is critical because it is a recurring cost. Vendors should be required to hold their support fees at the consumer price index. Maintenance fees below 20 percent of the software are considered below-market averages. Although vendors will discount maintenance and support, they are usually less flexible in this area because this is where they make their long-standing revenue.

5. **Recurring/transaction services costs.** Most systems use add-on services that can generate recurring fees, such as EDI services, eligibility, remittance, and electronic prescribing. Despite common beliefs, these services have a high mark-up value and can be negotiated at lower rates. In most cases, the vendor is reselling services from a third-party supplier who is providing the vendor with a kickback. This margin can come back to the customer in the form of a discount. Even though your vendor recommends a third-party supplier, you can still shop around for these services to find the best deal.

6. **Data conversion costs.** Although data conversions are usually a one-time fee, this service is almost always priced separately. Most vendors will agree to throw in a free conversion in exchange for buying the system. If the vendor is going to charge

your practice for this service, you should agree to pay only 50 percent up front and 50 percent after the conversion is fully verified.

7. **Interfacing costs.** Some vendors provide standard fixed-fee pricing for interfacing; others will provide custom pricing at your request. Similar to the data conversion service, many vendors will add interfacing as a purchase incentive. If the vendor is going to charge for this service, you should agree to pay only 50 percent up front and 50 percent after successful interfacing is verified. Vendors usually provide a 10 to 25 percent discount on interfacing.

CONCLUSION

Negotiation is a process of testing the other side's positions while knowing your own and representing yourself clearly and respectfully. The vendor will likewise be testing you by taking positions and assessing your responses.

As stated in Chapter 7, vendors like to offer special end-of-month, -quarter, or -year pricing to see if you will jump at these artificial deadlines. If you react to the offer, the vendor assumes you are in a hurry to do the deal without requesting concessions. Similarly, just as the vendor is testing your resolve, you need to test the vendor's positions by proposing your own terms, which will include "deal-breakers," absolute requirements, and terms that you want but are willing to give up—provided that you get some concessions in return.

A critical success factor during negotiation is the ability to a change a perception of the other with respect to what they will accept to close the deal. In short, the more the vendor believes that it has to make concessions before you will sign a contract, the greater the likelihood that the vendor will move closer toward more favorable terms and pricing for your practice. In this regard, your effectiveness in negotiations is dependent on whether you have credibly communicated your positions. Therefore, as much as you might like to abbreviate the negotiating process—particularly if you have an aversion to this form of exchange and communication—the best results are usually achieved after a prolonged period of negotiation in which (1) you are convinced that you have reached the vendor's "bottom line," and (2) the vendor is convinced that you will not go forward with the deal unless the terms meet your "bottom line."

The contract review process should include business and legal review by an outside expert who does not have any financial conflicts of interest. Although this chapter provides several examples of contract terms to negotiate, we recommend that you develop a list of all issues important to your practice to ensure nothing gets missed. Defining the potential issues and desired outcomes will help you navigate this process.

CHAPTER 9

Developing Your Project Budget

INTRODUCTION

Once vendor negotiations are complete, the next two steps in the conversion of your medical practice to electronic health records (EHRs) are developing a budget for the project and establishing an implementation plan. Chapter 10 will focus on developing your implementation plan, while we explore your project budget in this chapter.

Although certain aspects of financial planning for acquiring an EHR and some guidance have been provided on these topics in prior chapters, this chapter delves into the specifics. The goal is to institute a systematic financial work plan that will enable the practice to produce financial forecasts for the project.

This chapter also presents an implementation plan model that will help you set in motion each step of the project, ensuring a smooth and successful transition to EHR technology.

DEVELOPING A PROJECT BUDGET

The project budget is one of the most pivotal resources to any technology project. It encompasses considerable input and planning. Without it, there is no way to accurately trace spending and perform a return-on-investment (ROI) analysis of the project. A project budget can be used as a measuring stick to evaluate project performance. It can also assess how well thought out the project undertaking was overall.

In some cases, creating a project budget takes as long or even longer than actual project implementation. With an abundance of preparation and ample resources to determine the project's financial requirements, your practice will be able to determine the project's feasibility.

Putting Together a Budgeting Team

Budget creation should involve all of the project's stakeholders. These individuals have the responsibility to provide input and feedback when necessary. Without a project budget and the discipline to follow it, an organization can lose control of spending. Alternatively, with all stakeholders contributing to the budget document, the budget itself can serve as a useful governing document when making key financial decisions.

To start developing your project budget, begin by referring to the high-level budget that was drafted in the initial project stages. That draft budget is referred to as a *cost estimate*. It is an approximation of the financial impact of the project.

Alternatively, budgeting requires that project planners gather written estimates from potential partners and vendors. It is at this point that the participation of key on-staff stakeholders is crucial to developing a full understanding of the potential costs and resources associated with the project. Information technology (IT) managers, clinical staff, accounts receivable, human resources, executives, and other stakeholders should be brought together to contribute their knowledge to the budgeting and implementation process. Their expertise as subject matter experts (SMEs) is required to provide a realistic budget, obtain project buy-in, and, ultimately, establish accountability and momentum for the project.

Stakeholders perform research and analyze best practices for project implementation. They may call on vendors to provide a request for information for a product or service that will be developed as a resource for the project. In some projects, vendors may be considered stakeholders as well. Vendors can provide valuable insight into costs by quoting prices for potential solutions. Comparing multiple vendor quotes is a good way to assess where the value exists within the proposed product or service.

Developing a project budget should not involve re-creating the proverbial wheel. For example, citing information from similar projects can assist project planners in understanding the potential costs associated with the new project. Although each project is different, many technology-based projects contain similar components that can be used as points of reference. Team members can serve a valuable role by gathering ideas for costs. Project teams, sponsors, and others within your organization who have worked on similar projects can be of assistance in gathering information. Consulting with professionals who specialize in the task on which you are embarking will prove to be a valuable resource as well.

Labor and Materials

Dissecting your project plan will reveal the costs associated with labor and materials for each task. Total labor costs should include any tasks that require staff members to execute deliverables. Determine actual labor costs by applying labor rates to each detailed task. When tasks require the services of a physician, that physician's labor rate must be calculated in the budget. In addition, when the services of a licensed practitioner are required, the appropriate labor rate must be allocated for those tasks. In many cases, organizations do not have at their disposal all the necessary resources on hand. Budgeting for the cost to acquire project-based staff, whether long- or short-term, must be included in the project budget.

One cost that should not be overlooked is budget resources for project management. With a 2 percent increase from 2008 to 2009 (8.7 to 11.9 percent), the number of EHR implementations is increasing slowly.[1] This statistic is encouraging. However, with the deadline approaching for establishing a definition for the Meaningful Use criteria specified in the American Recovery and Reinvestment Act of 2009 (ARRA) and the Health Information Technology for Economic and Clinical Health Act (see Chapter 5 for details on Meaningful Use), having a seasoned EHR project management team on board can assist your practice in meeting time constraints for ARRA eligibility.

Hardware costs are also associated with certain tasks in the project schedule. Technology infrastructure components such as servers, routers, switches, wireless equipment, printers and scanners are common costs associated with EHR implementation. Lists of required and recommended hardware components should be requested when vendors submit their price quotes. These quotes should be reviewed and analyzed by IT subject matter experts (SMEs). Their feedback and suggestions should be duly noted. End users will often have hardware recommendations based on their personal preferences. Physicians, in most cases, will prefer one hardware manufacturer to another, and their opinions should be recognized. However, because compatibility issues may arise and drive up implementation costs, it is best to have all suggestions evaluated by IT SMEs to determine the effect of hardware purchases on the project budget.

Operating Costs

Ongoing operating costs should also be evaluated and documented in project budgets. The necessary rates for continuing operational costs associated with project delivery must be determined. Costs include but are not limited to networking (wide area and local area) costs, customer support costs, software licensing, lease or rental agreements and future service upgrades. Packaging solutions together from vendors can reduce costs, but this approach must be analyzed on a case-by-case basis. Server and systems hosting, network integration, and help desk support are all examples of managed service costs associated with ongoing operations of an EHR project.

Training and Travel

Categorize all other identifiable costs associated with a new project. Training and travel are often overlooked in the budgeting process. New technology solutions often involve training staff and business associates. In some cases, training can be performed on site by training consultants, but the travel expenses of these consultants typically need to be addressed in the project budget. In other cases, training simply cannot be performed on site and staff members may be required to travel. Either instance requires full review of potential travel costs.

Risk Assessment

Now that you have done the very best in working with stakeholders, vendors, staff, consultants, and solution providers to get the very best appraisal of the costs associated with the project, the next step is to measure risk. Risk assessment is also crucial to the success of a project budget. Crisis is inherent to every big project and problems always happen. How you plan for contingencies underlies the potential for success or failure in the project. Risk values should be added (padded) into cost assessments—and they are not to be considered sales inflation. Risk is always part of the price tag attached to new projects and it should be included in every budget. Risk line items should include experience of the project team, ability to support technology used, time shortages, the use of stationary vs. virtual teams, integration of third-party technology, the age of technology used, location of project manager and any unknown factors.

Once these risks have been identified, assign a percentage to each of them. For example, if you are integrating stand-alone practice management and EHR systems when your applications team has experience working with only one of the products, you would apply a risk percentage to that deliverable portion of the project. Another example would be the risk of delay in receiving hardware at your facility because of inclement weather or a natural disaster. The point is that, in terms of risk assessments, costs are not always measured in dollars and cents; they should be measured in time and human resources as well. When the focus is on financial cost instead of total value, there is a danger that, in the end, the costs will be higher than estimated because unrealistic milestones will not be met on schedule and more people will be needed to manage the project because software solutions are seen as too costly. Another example would be choosing a manual solution to adjust server usage instead of purchasing an automatic load balancer. Imagine having to manage each of the electrical circuits in your home so that you could use the clothes washing machine and automatic dishwasher at the same time. Yes, a circuit panel costs money and you must hire a trained electrician to install it, but what is gained in efficiency and safety is priceless.

BUDGET PROGRESSION

Project budgets are to be considered working documents. They require ongoing review and have a lifecycle of their own. The final project budget should be as accurate as possible and is derived from project estimates obtained at various stages of implementation. The *rough budget estimate* is the first edition of the budget and is drawn up in the initiation phase of the project lifecycle. The main purpose of the rough budget estimate is to draw interest of the organization to the project; it provides a quick view of the objectives, deliverables and a rough estimate of project costs for leaders. It has a range of variance from -25 to +75 percent accuracy.

The next version of the budget is the *contract estimate*. With a variance of accuracy ranging from -10 to +25 percent, the contract estimate is a more accurate version of the budget and is used later in the initiation phase of the project. It is expected to "drill down" into the project objectives and account for more detailed costs.

As mentioned earlier, data in these budget estimates can be gathered from previous project budgets, new research and input from stakeholders and other team members. The *definitive estimate* of the project budget is typically composed and concluded in the planning phase of the project. It accounts for details of all project costs, including labor, materials, operational and other tangible costs, and, of course, risk. It will be used throughout the project's lifecycle when actual costs must be known prior to making product purchases or payments for services. This budget is updated regularly, as soon as new information is available, and it is always under review to maintain control over project spending. This version of the budget has the highest amount of accuracy and generally has a variance of -5 to +10 percent for cost estimates.

Summary of Budgeting Process

An accurate project budget takes total team involvement and requires ongoing assessment of organizational needs and desires to fulfill project goals. The budget requires many changes throughout the project's lifecycle, and accuracy is improved as project planning advances. By analyzing labor, material, and operating and ongoing costs, the true cost of project implementation is revealed. Risk is a cost associated with the business of project management, and some risk value should be assigned to each project deliverable. A budget is essential to project success. Abiding by the budget provides a good foundation to analyze the project's return on investment.

CONCLUSION

This section has addressed an essential aspect of moving a medical practice from a paper-based office to an electronic operation. Planning and following a budget are foundational and fundamental to the timely and financially responsible execution of this ambitious goal.

REFERENCE

1. Jha AK, DesRoches CM, Kralovec PD, Joshi MS. A Progress Report on Electronic Health Records in U.S. Hospitals. Available at http://content.healthaffairs.org/content/early/2010/08/26/hlthaff.2010.0502.abstract. Accessed January 12, 2011.

CHAPTER 10

Developing Your Implementation Plan

INTRODUCTION

Following an implementation plan is essential for a medical practice to attain a successful transition to an electronic health record (EHR) system. Defining the project, establishing the governance, defining project scope and deliverables, instituting an implementation schedule, identifying project resources and managing stakeholders are vital aspects of a comprehensive implementation plan. By following the proven steps we outline in this chapter, your EHR project is more likely to reach a high degree of success.

PROJECT DEFINITION

The first step in developing an implementation plan is to define the project's scope. Although this is a simple or obvious step in concept, it requires significant time and attention. The definition of a project includes the following components: (1) why the organization is undertaking the project, (2) what the project intends to accomplish, (3) who will be involved in project execution, and (4) how the project will be executed. An example of an EHR project definition is as follows:

The goal of the General Hospital EHR project is to install, deploy, and implement the Acme EHR system at all hospital practices. Components to be included are as follows: messaging, electronic prescribing (E-prescribing), computerized practitioner order entry, and office note documentation. The system will interface with the following: local laboratory, local radiology department, and local pathology department. A patient portal will be available for appointment requests, patient registration, patient history, and communication with providers.

The guiding principles for the project are to: (1) improve patient safety and minimize medical errors; (2) improve access to patient data for quality-improvement projects; (3) improve patient access to providers; (4) present providers and staff with "just enough information, just in time" to improve provider and patient satisfaction; and (5) qualify for appropriate incentive programs.

The personnel assigned to this project are John Project Manager, Mary EHR App-Specialist, Dr. Jim Jones, Dr. Jane Champion, Joan Records Manager, Robert Nursing Manager, and Nick IT Manager. Gerry Compliance and Roger Billing will participate in the verification of clinical content. Help desk services will be outsourced to HelpDesk Ltd, which will be managed by Nick IT Manager. A physician advisory team composed of representative physicians from the practice will be consulted, as needed.

The system will be implemented using a phase-in approach by feature and functionality, as follows:

- Phase 1: Preload patient data
- Phase 2: Messaging, desktop management, and prescription refill management
- Phase 3: Point-of-care documentation by clinical site
- Phase 4: Provider orders and results management

One benefit of working in smaller practices is that decision making is often easier and more agile. However, in such settings, staff members will likely wear multiple "hats" when large projects are under way, such as EHR implementation. In addition, for smaller practices, it may be critical to augment current staffing levels with outside experts on occasion to ensure project success and reduce workflow and productivity interruptions.

Regardless of practice size, it is essential for EHR implementation teams to adopt project objectives that are clear, specific, measurable, achievable, and relevant—with a specific and realistic time frame attached to each project phase (see Table 10-1). Objectives help keep the EHR implementation team on track when the additional workload and pressure of the project take hold. The team can use these objectives to conduct formative evaluation of the project as it progresses. Objectives help the implementation

Objectives
Preload: Each staff member will successfully preload six patient medical records each day in Week One after the go-live date, working up to 15 medical records per day by Week Two.
Messaging: By the end of Week Two, all staff members will use internal messaging for laboratory and radiology studies that require insurance precertification.
Rx refill: 85% of refills on preloaded patient medical records will be completed using EHR and E-prescribing by the end of Week One. By the end of Week Four, 85% of all refills will be completed using EHR E-prescribing. (If the medical record has not been preloaded, staff will manually enter the requested medication to complete the refill request.)
Point-of-care documentation: Beginning at go-live, all office notes will be completed using the EHR; however, providers are permitted to dictate the history of the present illness.
Orders and results: Beginning at point-of-care documentation go-live, all provider orders will be placed using the EHR and all diagnostic test results will be viewed in the EHR. Paper results will no longer be available beginning in Week Three.

Table 10-1: Example EHR Implementation Plan Objectives

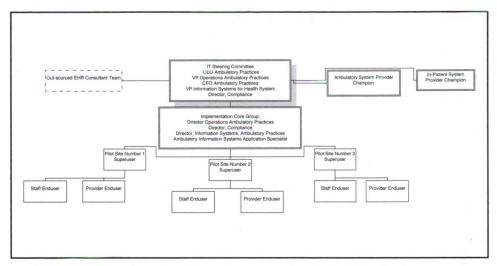

Figure 10-1: Example of an Organizational Chart for a Relatively Large Implementation Project

team measure the project's success and create opportunities to adjust the project plan as needed to build small achievements to successful implementation.

GOVERNANCE

Every major information technology (IT) implementation project runs a significant risk of failure. Health IT projects, because of their enormous complexity, are about as risky as such projects come. Governance plays a key role. Every project requires a clear and effective governance structure that includes a steering committee composed of key leadership or executive sponsors, such as the chief executive officer, chief information officer, chief financial officer, chief medical officer, and physician champions. The second "layer" of governance is the core implementation team. This second layer is more nimble and agile, completing the work of the EHR's file-build, content customization, workflow development, training, and support as each project phase goes live. Figure 10-1 is an example of an organizational chart for a relatively large EHR implementation project. As noted previously, it is typical in smaller practices for one person to fulfill multiple roles.

PROJECT SCOPE AND DELIVERABLES

Defining the project scope and deliverables early in project development and implementation helps prevent "scope creep" (i.e., the expansion of project deliverables). Once a new technology is introduced and catches on, it is very easy for additional functionalities to slip in, raising the danger that the implementation team may ignore critical elements that are central to the project's guiding principles. *Project scope* is the extent or range of the project and its deliverables. It includes measurable, tangible, and verifiable output, results, and items that must be produced to complete a project.

PROJECT RESOURCES

Project resources include financial support, leadership, and management as well as dedicated staff time for project implementation. Typically, project budgets are created when the decision to implement a project is made. A common pitfall in project development is not budgeting enough personnel for the project and making the project an additional responsibility for those already in place by job description. An EHR project needs the following personnel with dedicated project time:

- Physician/provider champion
- Project manager
- IT manager
- EHR application specialist
- Trainers
- "Super users"

Financial support for an EHR project is, of course, essential and must be realistic. Implementing an EHR project on a "shoestring budget" puts the project at risk for failure and extends the time needed for implementation and optimization.

The most neglected—and probably the most important—resource for successful EHR implementation is project support from practice leadership, both legitimate and apparent. Every practice has one provider to whom everyone looks for guidance and acceptance of changes. Support from this leader, and other workplace influencers, is foundational.

STAKEHOLDER MANAGEMENT

The first step is identifying project stakeholders and developing a plan that incorporates them. Because good EHR implementation and optimization affects every aspect of the practice, every staff member has a stake in the project's success. A common mistake among project planners is to ignore the role of billing and compliance staff in the success of the EHR. Although billing and compliance are not necessarily a focus of this project, they are a component of it and are necessary to review provider orders and diagnosis codes as well as the verification of clinical content.

Medical records staff are often fearful of losing their jobs as a result of the transition to EHRs. Although project implementation rarely decreases staffing immediately, it is important to consider how medical records staff can "retool" for the new system and fill a different role and function. Scanning and indexing are essential to the EHR adoption process, and work will be plentiful as long as paper continues to come into the practice.

Medical assistants and front desk staff may find that their roles expand with the use of EHR decision support applications. EHR systems encourage everyone to work up to their scope of practice. Front desk staff will now have access to each patient's EHR, allowing them to direct questions and schedule appointments more effectively. Furthermore, they can better monitor the flow of patients through the clinical area.

Although providers and nurses are the most prominent stakeholders in the EHR adoption process, it is important to remember that patients, too, are stakeholders. Unfortunately, during EHR implementation, patients are often an afterthought. Practices will learn that patients are generally pleased when their providers adopt EHR systems. They look forward to receiving better communication from the practice, more efficient management of their care, and faster service. That said, patients can be incorporated into the EHR implementation and optimization process simply by ensuring that staff communicates with them before, during and after the visit and by teaching providers to embrace, rather than ignore, computers in the examination rooms. Installing large monitors that can be easily viewed by the patient showing patient diagrams, radiology studies, and graphing progress on blood sugars and other lab results helps patients feel like full participants in their healthcare rather than helpless observers.

It is essential to include all stakeholders in EHR project planning and implementation—even, and perhaps especially, those who are resistant. In fact, you might find that initially resistant stakeholders can be the most effective in the selection and optimization processes because they are not blinded by a love of the technology and will be very honest about its flaws. That said, it is also important to manage stakeholder perceptions. Too often, the EHR implementation team is reactive, trying to make everyone happy. Change is difficult and does not occur without some disruption.

IMPLEMENTATION SCHEDULE

The implementation schedule should closely align with the following outline:
- Project phases
- Deliverable associated with each project phase
- Major activities required for each deliverable
- Key milestones
- Stakeholder responsible for delivery of each major activity
- Any dependencies

Typically, project phases for EHR adoption include building and deployment of technology infrastructure, system preload, messaging capabilities, E-prescribing applications, provider orders and results management, and, finally, point-of-care documentation. Project phases can also be broken down by clinical site (i.e., bringing all features and functionality live on a site-by-site basis). Another way to approach these project phases would be by provider or specialty. Regardless of the "roll-out" approach, the first phase of implementation requires addressing technology infrastructure.

A solid, reliable, robust technology infrastructure is critical to successful EHR project implementation. Therefore, addressing the technology infrastructure at the beginning of EHR implementation includes the following:
- Installation and build of the servers;
- Installation or redesign of the wide area network (links multiple sites) and the local area network (links multiple computers in one site);
- Purchase, configuration, and deployment of end-user hardware, such as thin client machines, personal computers (PC), tablet PCs, and/or laptops; and
- Deployment or remapping of printers and scanners.

Preloading patient data is an important and necessary implementation phase for several reasons. First, it is clear from research on IT adoption and assimilation that clinicians are more likely to use EHRs when pertinent clinical information is in the patient's medical record when they begin using it. Second, it gives staff an opportunity to practice navigating the system and entering data in a non-stressful environment, without a patient in front of them. Third, it moves structured data into the EHR, which can then be used for prescription refills, drug-to-drug and drug-to-allergy alerts, and populated problem lists.

Teaching staff how to use the system for messaging and E-prescribing is the next phase of the implementation plan. This phase provides some good features for communication regarding patient issues and is usually a "crowd pleaser" because E-prescribing is much easier than writing a prescription. E-prescribing is much faster for the patient as well.

Implementing electronic management of provider orders and diagnostic test results is, generally speaking, one of the more complex phases of the EHR implementation plan. This component of the plan should be started very early in the project because full integration with reference laboratories, radiology suites, and pathology laboratories is complicated and takes several cycles to complete. That said, viewing diagnostic test results and managing provider orders within the EHR system is much more efficient than paper management. It places all information at the provider's fingertips in a context that facilitates clinical decision making—so much so that we would discourage the purchase of any EHR system that does not offer this level of functionality. It is best to prioritize the most critical interfaces, making them a requirement for go-live. As with other features, staff should plan to work toward optimizing integration over time.

The final phase of the implementation plan is point-of-care documentation. This phase of the project requires the most behavior modification from providers. At this phase of implementation, the provider is now using the EHR at the point of care with patients present. He/she is documenting the patient visit for the medical record and satisfying compliance requirements for billing. Most providers are accustomed to dictating physician notes for each patient visit; they often struggle with the transition—pointing and clicking in templates to provide documentation. This phase requires tremendous amounts of planning because clinical content must be prepared for customized forms. We recommend that customization be kept to a minimum initially, at least until the provider is comfortable with the logic of the new system and understands how the forms are designed to function. Selecting a system with robust content for the practice specialty makes this process easier on everyone.

Once all phases of the EHR system are live, the practice shifts into system review. EHR systems require ongoing review and optimization using a structured process for change management. It is at this time that the EHR team evolves into a health information management committee. The new committee includes representatives from providers, nursing staff, clinic operations, medical records, compliance and billing, at a minimum. If there is a quality assurance officer and/or a risk manager in the organization, those individuals should also be included.

CONCLUSION

Admittedly, transitioning a practice to an EHR system is difficult. However, this recommended model for implementation ensures that your practice has its best opportunity for a successful transition to EHR technology. As this chapter indicates, participation and support from many individuals, including stakeholders, are the foundation for achieving the practice's full transition.

CHAPTER 11

EHR Optimization

INTRODUCTION

Optimal use of electronic health records (EHRs) requires adopting a plan for continuous quality improvement. EHRs are a good example of today's "disruptive innovations" in healthcare. EHRs have a role in revolutionizing healthcare delivery. That said, we have a long way to go—as EHR end users, as an industry in terms of what EHRs can and cannot do, and as a nation of patients who will soon have real-time access to our health information anytime, anywhere.

The EHR of the future will support smartphone technology; allow emergency medical personnel to access personal health information when treating an unconscious patient; allow specialists to "see" patients regardless of the geographic location of either party; and ensure all patients with a particular disease process receive the very best "gold standard" care, regardless of where they live or their socioeconomic standing. EHRs will seamlessly integrate the presentation of health information to just the right people at just the right time across transitions of care, allowing for minimal delay in treatment.

Optimal means using something in the best possible way. When speaking of EHRs, *optimization* combines quality improvement initiatives with the power of the technology to directly improve patient care. The first step in optimization is to recognize the need for ongoing development of the EHR by the practice. Until recently, many (if not most) EHR systems were used to house and distribute dictation. EHRs are not widely used in medical practices, which has limited product development. However, more widespread use of these systems will certainly encourage vendors to develop systems that are more user friendly; easier to install, implement, and maintain; and include more features and functionality. We explore in this chapter the many ways to optimize EHRs.

MAKING THE MOST OF AVAILABLE TECHNOLOGY

There are a variety of areas to focus on for EHR optimization, such as patient kiosks and portals, electronic messaging, interfaces, document imaging, fax servers, and data management.

Patient Kiosks

Kiosks allow patients to register and maintain accurate demographic information for the practice. Accurate demographic information is the first step in the revenue cycle and leads to compressed and reliable cash cycles for the practice. Kiosks also improve collections. Most kiosk applications are equipped with credit card swiping capabilities and will not fail to ask patients to pay overdue balances.

In addition, kiosks allow patients to review and enter data without interacting with front desk staff. It offers an abbreviated patient check-in process that improves practice throughput, reduces patient wait time, improves patient and provider satisfaction and allows improved productivity for front desk staff. Even if only half of the practice's patients check in using the kiosk, a considerable amount of front desk staff hours are freed up for other tasks. Although patient kiosks represent a significant hardware investment for the practice, they also represent a significant return on investment.

Patient Portal

Patient portals are no longer a luxury; they are becoming a requirement. The final Meaningful Use (MU) criteria states that medical practices must be capable of the following:

> Provide patients with timely electronic access to their health information (including lab results, problem list, medication list, medication allergies) within four business days of the information being available to the EP. *Additional Information:* Information that must be provided electronically is limited to that information that exists electronically in or is accessible from the certified EHR technology and is maintained by or on behalf of the EP. At a minimum, certified EHR technology makes available lab test results, problem list, medication list, and medication allergy list.[1]

Although patient portals are not one of the mandatory criteria described in the final rules for the American Recovery and Reinvestment Act of 2009 (ARRA), it is listed as one of five optional criteria from which the practice must choose. In addition, a practice may choose to make patient data available online to meet one of the optional criteria described in the final rules for ARRA.

Many patient portals allow patients to update their medical and surgical histories online, communicating directly with the EHR. Usually, patient-entered information is available for import by practice staff after it has been reviewed and deemed accurate. Only then is it permanently imported into the patient's medical record. In addition, most portal applications can be configured to allow patients to schedule appointments, request medication refills or referrals, and to request communication with the practice regarding health-related concerns or billing. In turn, the practice can communicate electronically, eliminating the inevitable phone tag that occurs when trying to reach patients by telephone. Patient self-access to medical records reduces staff time devoted to basic release-of-information requests. All these functions improve the patient-provider relationship by encouraging patient engagement in healthcare decisions and health maintenance.

In addition, patient portals represent a new opportunity for practices to communicate with their patients. Portals allow access to asynchronous communication with providers and nurses. Portals also allow a practice to reach out to patients for various health-promotion and disease-prevention activities (e.g., influenza vaccinations, mammograms, annual gynecologic examinations, prostate health examinations, chronic disease management activities).

Patient portals also allow for direct electronic communication with other local providers who would otherwise not have access to a patient's medical record. Often, the portal will have a secure messaging component that can be used, with the patient's permission, to distribute protected health information to other health professionals when consultation with specialists is required, for example.

Electronic Messaging

All certified EHR products support electronic messaging among providers and staff in a given practice. In most cases, it is very difficult during project implementation to eliminate the paper cues used in a practice. When optimizing the use of the EHR, practices should look for opportunities to eliminate paper and use real-time electronic messaging as the primary means of communicating. This switch is particularly useful in practices with multiple sites because it allows communication to happen across various sites and transitions of care. In addition, electronic messaging can be configured in such a way as to allow for work to continue when staff is on vacation or out sick. Out-of-office replies can often be applied and proxy desktops configured so that referral requests always go to a referral proxy that can be monitored and managed by staff. Using phone notes to document phone calls with patients allows for replies to be tracked and documented in the medical record.

Interfaces

Technology interfaces reduce the amount of paper coming into a practice. They also reduce the need for scanning and indexing even as they improve care coordination and system usefulness for providers. Interfacing is not easy, however, and although EHR systems are maturing, the ability of disparate systems to communicate remains somewhat crude. Practices should work with local hospital systems, laboratory and radiology vendors, and other sources for referral/referring functions to develop a health information exchange plan that is continuously and consistently optimized. They should also seek interfacing partners that add value, such as advanced beneficiary notice verification at the point of care, provider order auto-completion once test results are available, and data dictionary management when laboratories and radiology centers change/update coding. Paper hospital stay documents, such as discharge summaries, emergency room documentation, and operative notes should be treated as signed documents via an interface system to eliminate duplicate work for providers.

Interfaces also improve laboratory and radiology utilization by providing a complete order at the point of care. Many provider order interfaces include advanced beneficiary notice verification, which improves denials management. In addition, they can often manage the "ask-at-order-entry questions" such as dietary fasting requirements, chronic conditions that affect contrast radiology dye administration, and right vs. left side for basic radiograms. Asking these questions and ensuring the patient understands the instructions provided saves healthcare dollars by ensuring the correct test is ordered and can be performed when scheduled. Sending provider orders across an interface is challenging and requires that the laboratory is capable of receiving orders from disparate EHR systems.

That said, there is real value to computerized practitioner order entry (CPOE). CPOE requires physicians to provide a diagnosis or identify symptoms at the point of care while ordering tests to either confirm or manage the diagnosed condition. Although CPOE requires providers to input structured data, the order is now available for tracking in the system where results are available electronically and insurance is billed directly. Furthermore, all parties are assured that the conditions for medical necessity will be met because the provider has diagnosis-specific point-of-care decision support. The tracking features of CPOE interfaces ensure that patients follow through on ordered diagnostic tests and that results are received. The feature also helps to improve patient compliance with routine screening and diagnostics for chronic disease management. Finally, until direct order entry is available, CPOE ensures a legible printed requisition is available as a reminder to the patient and for subsequent use by the laboratory.

Document Imaging

A key function to optimize is document imaging. Many EHR vendors incorporate a document imaging system that allows for automatic document indexing and the management of discreet data. Most practices launching a new EHR system will use document management to transition paper medical records to EHRs and to manage the paper documents that continue to come into the practice. Furthermore, many items are more easily handled on paper and will continue to remain in that format. Most practices in the late stages of implementation understand how difficult it is to stay ahead of the work of manual indexing for paper documents.

Practices should consider adding plug-in software that would allow document rules to be built so that certain paper documents are automatically stored in patient EHRs. This software typically allows discreet data to be pulled from scanned documents to populate the patient EHRs. Examples include dates for routine screenings (e.g., pap smear, mammogram, prostate health screening). Often test results can also be extracted as discreet data, allowing the practice to more efficiently track the results of preventive screening.

Maximizing Fax Server

Fax servers are great time savers that provide a very efficient way of distributing patient information and results to referral/referring providers. Fax servers eliminate the need to print and fax paper, including prescriptions (i.e., for pharmacies that do not accept electronic prescribing). Fax servers also allow incoming faxes to be distributed directly to a patient's EHR with provider inbox notification. That said, fax servers must be correctly configured to fulfill these functions so staff can easily distribute provider notifications.

Managing Data

Managing patient data to help providers improve healthcare quality by inviting patients in for preventive health services and/or management of chronic disease is a productive use of EHR optimization as well as practice time and energy. Many practices struggle with using data to address quality-of-care issues because providers often dispute data accuracy. The first step in this quality-improvement process is demonstrating to clinicians how the data is collected, mined, and reported. Doing so will help staff gain provider buy-in to the data's accuracy. After everyone agrees the data is as accurate as possible and acknowledges that all new data is entered by providers at the point of care through CPOE, honest discussion on quality issues can ensue.

At a recent user conference for a leading EHR vendor, one presenter related a story of using data to drive the quality of care for all diabetic patients in a practice. He described the long road to convincing everyone the data was accurate. Once that hurdle was achieved, the group learned that all diabetic patients with a hemoglobin A1c higher than 9 (below 6 is considered acceptable) were not receiving the "gold standard" of care—prescribed insulin. This realization allowed clinicians to improve the standard of care for diabetic patients in their practice. By providing better and more reliable care for all of their diabetic patients, the practice ultimately improved their patients' quality of life and saved healthcare delivery dollars because they were preventing potential complications that are very expensive to treat. Powerful stuff!

Another advantage of gathering patient data is the ability of the practice to improve provider utilization and production by initiating and tracking preventive care services. Additional provider encounters of this kind teach patients how to best use healthcare, saving healthcare dollars by preventing serious illness or disease complications while also providing practice revenue.

MANAGEMENT OF INFORMATION SYSTEMS

For early adopters of health information technology (IT), managing the various systems and infrastructure for EHRs has undoubtedly been challenging. In many cases, the practice's tech savvy physician has been managing, updating, troubleshooting and optimizing the EHR. The optimization phase is a good time to review workload optimization. Is EHR management a good use of physician time? Would it be more cost-effective for the practice to hire IT staff or outsource technology management? Is technology being fully used by the practice and its providers? If not, would better technology management improve IT utilization and reduce costs? What will it take for a practice to reach the government's Meaningful Use requirements? Does the practice have the necessary staff in terms of time and skill to participate fully in stimulus incentive programs?

As noted previously, early adopters (both vendors and clients) will have to address the new Meaningful Use guidelines as part of their optimization efforts (see Chapter 5). Many of the goals in the new guidelines,[2] which are directed at improving quality, safety, and efficiency, are dependent on electronic tracking of common health measures that are essential to primary care medicine. Alternatively, many specialists (e.g., ophthalmology, dermatology) do not routinely capture blood pressure measurements, height, weight, or body mass index because that data is not clinically relevant to the care they deliver. The final rules indicate that specialists who do not routinely collect certain data report the numerator and denominator as zero.[2]

CONCLUSION

EHR optimization is a process that continues throughout the life of an EHR application. Planning for optimization or "full ownership" of the EHR by the organization is a critical factor in achieving success. Many practices make the mistake of under-resourcing the ongoing maintenance and development of EHRs. Implementation is only the beginning. The goal is total assimilation of the EHR in the practice.

REFERENCES

1. CMS. Medicare & Medicaid EHR Incentive Program, Eligible Professional Meaningful Use Menu Set Measures 5 of 10, Stage 1, November 7, 2010. www.cms.gov/EHRIncentivePrograms/Downloads/5PatientElectronicAccess.pdf. Accessed January 21, 2011.

2. Blumenthal D. *N Engl J Med.* Aug 5, 2010;363:501-504. http://www.nejm.org/doi/full/10.1056/NEJMp1006114. Accessed January 12, 2011.

CHAPTER 12

Lessons Learned

INTRODUCTION

Medical practices are experiencing more pressure than ever to implement electronic health records (EHRs). Fortunately, they are experiencing more incentives than ever before for participation as well. Meaningful Use EHR adoption incentives allow medical practices to offset the significant financial costs of installation and implementation. In addition, EHRs allow groups that perform electronic prescribing (E-prescribing) and those that efficiently and effectively collect data on quality indicators to obtain financial incentives from the Centers for Medicare & Medicaid Services (CMS). Private insurers are also following the lead of CMS to improve the presence of EHRs in ambulatory care practice. Clearly, there is a growing recognition that high-quality, efficient patient care is cost effective and will save healthcare dollars.

The goals of using EHRs include improving the quality and safety of patient care and care coordination while encouraging patient and family engagement in the healthcare decision-making process. It is hoped that these improvements in health connectivity will translate into improved national health. Unlike paper medical records, optimized EHRs are capable of doing much more than storing documentation of office encounters. In addition to supporting practice workflow, EHRs help with post-encounter task management, such as tracking provider orders and results, referrals, and E-prescribing; follow-up patient communications; charting and graphing patient care longitudinally; and passing patient charges directly to the billing system. In brief, EHRs are better than paper medical records because they have to be; they require a tremendous investment of time and money from a practice.

This chapter summarizes lessons learned from numerous EHR implementation projects, including theories on change management.

FIFTEEN STEPS

Surveys tell us that although 25 to 30 percent of all physicians report purchasing and "using" EHRs, most are not using the systems as they are designed or intended to be used. We are learning that, of those who have invested in EHR technology, only 5 to 10 percent of physicians are making full use of EHRs. This lack of EHR absorption makes their return on investment (ROI)—and, more importantly, return on objective (i.e., the objectives now defined by meaningful use criteria)—low and unfavorable.

In this chapter, we share 15 steps that, when followed by physicians and other providers, enhance a practice's opportunity for EHR success. Although none of these steps is particularly easy, you will find that when they are followed you will have an EHR-integrated practice that has the power to transform healthcare delivery, making it more effective, less expensive, and more enjoyable for all parties.

1. **Mentally prepare everyone for the demands of EHR implementation.** Prepare providers, staff and yourself to learn something new. None of us is very comfortable in this role, but becoming a learner is the critical first step to ensuring success. Experience tells us that this challenge can be especially difficult for physicians precisely because they are extremely competent in the examination room caring for patients and have grown comfortable conducting business using paper medical records and dictation. The EHR is a completely new way of using clinical data to care for patients. Groups successful with EHR implementation cite the need for practices to make a firm commitment to clinical transformation.

2. **Prepare the patients for EHR implementation.** The vast majority of patients perceive the move to EHRs as a positive step for the practice and for them as individual patients. However, it is important to continue addressing security and privacy issues. Using a slogan like "We are slowing down now so we can speed up later" engages patients in the process of implementation and gives them fair warning that the first few visits after the go-live date might take a bit more time to complete.

3. **Ensure the implementation team is well supported.** In most cases, the EHR team is extremely dedicated and committed to a successful implementation process, including thorough assimilation into the practice. It is critically important that they have the resources they need to ensure success. Just as providers know more about medicine and healthcare provision, the team knows more about planning EHR implementation. Teams often work very hard at refining workflow models and adjusting workloads only to be stopped in their tracks by provider resistance. Encouraging provider involvement along the way mitigates "eleventh-hour" problems. EHRs require sponsorship at the highest levels of the organization.

4. **Focus on value, not cost.** The most expensive EHR is the one that sits on the shelf. The EHR implementation team needs an adequate budget that is focused on value. ROI will be achieved quickly with everyone participating and supporting project goals. "Catch up" will be required if the practice's information technology (IT) infrastructure has not had adequate investment and attention through the years. IT must be a line item on the annual budget and receive continual investment, especially once a practice decides to convert to EHRs.

5. **Stay positive, especially in front of staff.** There is no doubt that the process of launching a new EHR system is difficult and will generate some frustration. However, it is important to keep in mind the principle that frustration can be either an asset—helping to move the process along in a way that works best for the practice—or a hindrance, stopping the project in its tracks. When making a

fundamental change like EHR implementation, expect frustration and try to use it to move the process forward. Resisting frustration makes the process more difficult, but using it to motivate providers and staff to learn the system—adapting to new features and functionality—will make the process easier and more effective, reducing the time to achieve ROI.

6. **Commit to learning the system incrementally.** It is overwhelming to learn a new comprehensive EHR system all at once. The implementation team should be dedicated to a phased-in, incremental approach to system integration. They should present providers and staff with the opportunity to learn the system one or two features at a time. Learning each feature slowly and completely in this manner will increase system integration and shorten the learning curve. Another consequence of this incremental approach is a growing understanding of the system's logic. Understanding the EHR system's logic helps providers and staff be better prepared to participate in the customization process during system optimization.

7. **Decreasing patient volume during implementation is essential for success.** The process of implementing a new EHR system is a "pay me now or pay me later" situation where productivity trade-offs are involved. Decreasing patient volume modestly during each phase of the project gives providers and staff an atmosphere and environment that are more conducive to learning and assimilating the system into the fabric of the practice. Reducing patient volume initially provides the added benefit of allowing the practice to more quickly, reliably, and confidently return to full patient volumes later. Decreased patient volume must be added to project budget projections. Based on our experience, when all is said and done, this deferred patient volume usually has the same effect as an additional week of vacation time per provider.

8. **Show the system early and often.** All members of the implementation team should be equipped with access to the system so they can demonstrate system features and functionality frequently to providers and staff. Workflow development must be done within the context of the system and can only be done properly by "running" the work flow with the system in mock trials.

9. **Incorporate stakeholders throughout implementation.** When in doubt, ask. Show the system and illustrate how the team intends to address implementation details. Identify all stakeholders. The EHR system will affect every aspect of the practice, from providers, nursing, and front desk staff to scheduling, billing, and medical records staff. Remember to include telephone triage staff and staff in charge of referrals and prior authorization. Taking the time to show the system to staff at regular intervals has the benefit of allowing you to communicate project progress, assuring staff that they will be well prepared to use the product in the clinic.

10. **Take training seriously.** Training is an opportunity to be a learner, ask questions and gain a practical understanding of the system. It is critical that providers and clinic staff attend the training sessions offered to them. The implementation team should be committed to providing several training options. In addition, though this advice may be obvious, it is critical that the EHR team is in the office for the

go-live date for additional support and training. It is well known that training "at the elbow" of end users is the most effective for task retention.

11. **Offer classroom and at-the-elbow training options.** As noted above, at-the-elbow training can be very effective. That said, some providers may be disappointed by what the system can and cannot do but, mainly, by how much different it is from paper medical records. When working at the elbow of providers, avoid responding to their questions by saying, "The system cannot do that." Instead, try listening to the provider to determine what they are actually trying to do. Using the phrase "Help me understand the problem you are trying to solve" can be effective.

12. **Take medical record preloading seriously.** Preloading data from paper medical records is an opportunity for the practice to get codified, discreet patient data into the system. Generally, preloading consists of manually transferring problem and medication lists, allergies, and immunization histories into the EHR system along with scanned diagnostic reports, surgical reports, etc. A secondary goal is for staff to experience working with the system independent of patient visits. Providers who commit to preloading at least three complete medical records per week are typically more successful in integrating the EHR into their practice.

13. **Using the system, enter at least five patient encounters before the go-live date.** Using the system to enter a completed patient encounter gives the provider more experience with the system and allows him/her to identify potential areas for customization that will improve workflow and efficiency.

14. **Require providers and staff to commit to using the system as taught consistently for the first 28 days after go-live.** The pathway to successful use of EHR follows the classic novice-to-expert trajectory. At the beginning of implementation, providers and staff will be very focused on the technology—learning how to incorporate the use of a computer in the patient visit, learning how to navigate the system, and learning where to find vital patient information. As EHR fluency increases, the technology becomes second nature. The novice phase of EHR assimilation can be shortened by regular, disciplined use of the system for the first 28 days—the amount of time most experts say is required to learn new behaviors.

15. **Commit to ongoing system development—and the change management process.** Go-live is just the beginning of EHR implementation and assimilation. As the practice becomes more familiar with how the EHR works and what is possible within it, there needs to be a formal process in place to submit changes and continually improve the system. Keeping the implementation team intact is a good way to begin the optimization process. Establishing a health information management committee is the ultimate goal. This committee will function in a manner similar to a hospital's forms committee, which manages how information is entered and maintained in paper medical records. The new health information management committee should be comprised of the EHR application manager and providers as well as risk management, medical records, and compliance specialists. The critical element is ensuring that staff knows how to make changes to clinical content and workflow. Evaluating how the system is being used is essential. A good tool is the HIMSS Analytics EMR Adoption Model,[SM] which scores

hospitals in the HIMSS Analytics Database on their progress in completing the eight stages (0 to 7) to creating a paperless patient record environment. Information is available at www.himssanalytics.org/hc_providers/emr_adoption.asp.

CONCLUSION

Implementing and integrating the EHR will touch every part of an ambulatory care practice. It is and should remain a transformational process. It is critical, particularly for physician owners, to allow implementation staff to guide and lead this process. Technology, workflow, content and training must be addressed in each project phase to ensure that the transformation is complete and the EHR does not become a very expensive, digitized paper medical record. To be successful in EHR integration, physicians and other providers must be willing to submit to the process and allow themselves to be novices again.

Chapter 13

Future Trends

INTRODUCTION

Our ever-changing healthcare system and the information technology (IT) supporting it guarantee only one thing: continual evolution that includes new technology and policies. As a result, trends often emerge as a way to prepare for the future and as an alternative to the status quo as the technology improves to address current challenges. Trends often emerge out of several areas, not just gadgets and devices. In fact, policy trends often create opportunity for new technologies to develop. For example, after the 1996 passage of the Health Insurance Portability and Accountability Act (HIPAA), an entire industry of solutions was created to address new privacy and security laws. After the terrorist attacks on September 11, 2001, new security rules created another industry which comprises security consulting, devices and network traffic monitoring. The popularity of the Internet also generated new trends. Before the Internet, the need for antivirus software did not exist. Internet service providers and, more recently, social networking sites were all born out of Internet technology.

This chapter addresses future trends in the five areas: (1) policy, (2) integration and interoperability, (3) new technologies, (4) software, and (5) social networking.

POLICY

Policies have been included as a trend in this context as a result of the enormous flood of new policies and agencies overseeing health IT adoption. Although we will not cover every such policy, in the past five years these policies have been some of the fastest emerging trends in the healthcare system and more developments continue to evolve every day. Some policies, such as HIPAA, may seem neither current nor even a trend; however, ramifications from its passage continue to evolve. In fact, many elements of HIPAA were updated/modified with the passage of the American Recovery and Reinvestment Act of 2009 (ARRA). Here are some of the most notable policies created during the past fifteen years:

- **HIPAA.** The Office for Civil Rights enforces the HIPAA privacy rule, which protects the privacy of individually identifiable health information. The privacy rule provides federal protections for personal health information held by covered entities and gives patients an array of rights with respect to that information. The privacy rule is balanced so that it permits the disclosure of personal health information needed for patient care and other important purposes. It is anticipated that HIPAA will continue to play a large role in healthcare and that it will likely come back to the forefront of our attention as the trend toward electronic health records (EHRs) continues. There is likely to be additional regulatory guidance regarding how healthcare providers manage and treat electronic patient data, including how we store and protect it.

- **The Healthcare Information Technology Standards Panel.** This panel was the result of a cooperative partnership between the public and private sectors. It was formed for the purpose of harmonizing and integrating IT standards to meet clinical and business needs for sharing electronic information among organizations and systems. This cooperation is an important policy trend because public-private integration is still evolving and maturing. There are also several groups and solutions emerging to deal with integration demand.

- **Healthcare reform.** Healthcare reform is expected to usher in a new era in medicine, which will have an impact on health IT. Although the full breadth of this impact is currently unknown, health IT is expected to be a centerpiece. For example, accountable care organizations (ACOs) are emerging as a result of healthcare reform. ACOs are designed around value-based compensation and compensation that is based on patient outcomes. Health IT will be critical to aggregate multiple caregivers and data elements to achieve success under this model. Health IT is also expected to eliminate waste in administrative functions, such as manual paperwork processing. See Table 13-1 for a complete list of industry and organization standards.

INTEGRATION AND INTEROPERABILITY

The trend toward health IT integration arose as soon as it was realized how difficult and expensive it was/is to interface multiple IT solutions. In the early 1990s, most EHRs were sold as stand-alone systems, a single solution database operating on a single server without third-party integration of any kind. However, it soon became apparent that these systems needed to be interfaced with practice management systems.

In some cases, these interfaces were never developed and systems operated independently, creating labor duplications and inefficiencies. As a result, a trend toward enterprise (fully integrated solutions with practice management and EHR components) or single vendor (solutions operating on a single database supplied by one vendor) solutions emerged. This shift toward interoperability inspired a trend toward mergers and acquisitions among the vendors, creating an entirely new market of vendors and solutions for healthcare. Many new vendors were building products on a single database. Merging vendors began developing a single brand and embedding integration for acquired products. Next, an entirely new industry of vendors and solutions began developing products to aggregate data-sharing repositories among caregivers. These are the vendors that now typically provide software to health information exchanges (HIE) or community health records, where there is a need to connect data from several caregivers into a single repository.

Accredited Standards Committee (ASC)
ASCX 12; ASC X3; ASC X Z80
American College of Radiology National Electrical Manufacturers Association (ACR-NEMA)
American Dental Association for Accredited Standards Committee MD156
American Society for Testing and Materials (ASTM)
Accredited Standards Organization (ASO)
Health Level Seven - HL7
Clinical Context Object Workgroup (CCOW)
Institute of Electrical & Electronic Engineers (IEEE)
National Council for Prescription Drug Programs (NCPDP)
ANSI Healthcare Information Standards Board (HISB)
The Systematized Nomenclature of Medicine - College of American Pathologists (SNOMED)
International Organization for Standardization (ISO)
American National Standards Institute (ANSI)
International Telegraph & Telephone Consultative Committee (CCITT)
Committee European De Normalization (CEN)
U.S. Government (HHS, HCFA, FDA, AHCPR, GAO, NIST, NBS and others)
Joint Healthcare Information Technology Alliance (JHITA) including AHIMA, HIMSS, AMIA
Health Industry Manufacturers Association (HIMA)
American Nursing Association and other clinical professional societies
Computer-based Patient Record Institute (CPRI)
Medical Records Institute (MRI)
Workgroup for Electronic Data Interchange (WEDI)

Table 13-1: Industry and Organizations Standards

The word *interoperability*, which defines the ability of diverse systems and organizations to work together to share information, began to be used as one of the descriptions for getting systems to communicate with one another, with a goal of eventually having everyone connected. Trends towards integration and interoperability continue to evolve because connecting to regional HIEs under ARRA is a requirement for practices to qualify for financial stimulus incentives. It is expected that many states/commonwealths will develop their own HIEs. Alternatively, regional HIEs will arise. Both types of HIE will be required to conform to the standards specified by the Nationwide Health Information Network (www.hhs.gov/healthit/healthnetwork/background/). Eventually, all HIEs will be interconnected to allow for the nationwide exchange of clinical information among caregivers, payers, and consumers. Deadlines for HIE completion are currently unknown, but experts predict it will take a considerable amount of time to overcome patient privacy concerns and to address existing patient privacy policies to maintain nationwide data integrity.

TECHNOLOGIES

One of the more exciting trends in healthcare is the evolution of technologies and devices. Devices have been improving dramatically during the past several decades, and in almost every case, as the technology improves, costs goes down. You may have heard of the term *Moore's Law*, which was coined based on an observation by Gordon Moore (cofounder of Intel Corporation) that the number of transistors on a microprocessor would double periodically (approximately every 18 months). He made this famous comment in 1965 when there were approximately 60 such devices on a microprocessor chip. Proving the accuracy of Moore's Law, four decades later, Intel placed 1.7 billion transistors on its Itanium chip. This law (or prediction) has been widely proven true, although the time frame has been lengthened to 24 months and is predicted to level out in 2015. One area where this rapid increase in quality and decrease in price has been most clearly visible is in entertainment devices, most especially music players. In 1954, the first portable transistor radio was released, followed soon by the turntable, then the eight-track tape player, the cassette player, the CD player, and now digital music, which is generally stored on MP3 players the size of a credit card with no moving parts.

Healthcare is no different, especially in the use of technology to operate medical practices. In fact, not long ago, many practices managed their billing and patient balances on paper index cards or on a system called a "peg board."

In the early 1980s, desktop personal computers (PCs) began to appear, but they were bulky, slow, and expensive, with limited functionality. Today's desktop PCs are much smaller, more powerful, and less expensive. Even now, desktop PCs are starting to become obsolete as more people move exclusively to laptop computers and tablet PCs.

The current trend emerging for gadgets is what are known as mobile devices or handheld computers. Although personal digital assistants (PDAs) have been around for years, they are now evolving into much more, and they come in all shapes and sizes. For example, a smartphone is both a cellular phone and a PDA and it can run software applications and browse the Internet. Most recently, we have started to see the development of mini-notebook computers and devices like the iPad, which are completely driven by touch screen technology. These personal computing devices have decreased in size and increased in power through the years, and they are increasingly being used at the point of care as a result of improving data synchronization.

In the past, the biggest concern many had regarding personal computing via handheld devices was about the amount of data such a device could store. The threat of losing the device or having it stolen was enough to discourage widespread use. However, now that most of these devices are capable of accessing data remotely, no data is stored on the device itself. In addition, data is encrypted when it is transferred, making it safe for transmittal and avoiding the issue of data being out of sync with the primary server.

SOFTWARE

Trends in software are seen in two main areas. The first of these is the development of products and tools intended to enhance or augment existing EHR systems, such as personal health records, patient kiosks, and electronic data interchange services. The second is a trend in how we acquire software.

Software Development

Descriptions of several trends in software development follow:

- **Personal health records (PHRs).** Although PHRs are not entirely new, they are beginning to reemerge with the recent passage of healthcare reform. Some experts believe that accountability for healthcare outcomes among consumers and physicians will become more prominent. To this end, tools such as PHRs will be required to allow patients to electronically store and manage their own health information. Both Google and Microsoft Corporation have developed PHRs that are free to the consumer.

- **Patient kiosks.** Similar to the self-service terminals at airports and grocery stores, patient kiosks are appearing at physician practices. As addressed in Chapter 10, kiosks that are available for patient check-in can collect information about the visit without front desk staff involvement. Likewise, kiosks can be used to take patient copayments. Proponents of patient kiosks argue that these tools collect data more accurately and consistently than staff. For example, a kiosk will never forget to ask a patient for money. Kiosk skeptics argue that elderly patients may find these devices difficult to use. Skeptics also note that there could be some sanitary issue drawbacks to these machines when numerous sick patients use the same touch screen—though few have raised this point with regard to pen use for traditional clipboard sign-ins. Medical practices will always have some threats regarding the spread of illness. That said, these devices seem to be growing in popularity.

- **Patient portals.** A patient portal is similar to the PHR except that the practice owns and manages this tool, using it to assist with patient communication. The scope of these tools can be rather limited, allowing patients only to view and print their records online, or they can be rather expansive, offering interactive solutions that allow for online bill paying, e-consultations, appointment scheduling, and secure patient-provider messaging. A patient portal is one requirement for medical practices to qualify for financial stimulus incentives as designated under ARRA and The Health Information Technology for Economic and Clinical Health Act—although guidelines are still being defined. Portal proponents feel that these tools empower patients and provide an additional method of patient-physician communication. They argue that patient portals also reduce practice costs by allowing patients to manage their own medical records instead of calling the practice to request copies or to ask questions about test and laboratory results. Portal skeptics feel that these tools create risks to patient privacy. Although patient data is not exchanged and each patient has a unique sign-on (i.e., login and password), there is always a risk of a privacy violation. However, because most third-party payers do not compensate physicians for online consultations, adoption of this technology has been relatively slow.

- **HIE tools.** As noted above, HIEs are emerging as a way to connect caregivers. Accordingly, new software vendors and products are emerging to manage these transactions.
- **Mobile applications.** With the growing popularity of smartphones and mobile devices such as the iPad, there is a growing trend toward developing software applications that will run native on these devices. A native application is one that is specifically designed to run on a device's operating system and machine firmware. Typically, it needs to be adapted for different devices. A "Web app", or Internet browser application, is one in which all or some parts of the software are downloaded from the Web each time it is run.[1]

Software Acquisition and Delivery

Next are several new trends in how software is being acquired and delivered. Table 13-2 shows the evolutionary course of software acquisition and delivery.

Currently, software as a service (SaaS) is a popular trend because medical practices often do not have the IT resources necessary on-site to manage complicated EHR systems. SaaS is appealing because it is a subscription-based service, usually requiring no up-front investment. As for drawbacks, the practice never owns the EHR system. It is a situation analogous to renting a house; you never own it but you are also not responsible for any of the upkeep or management issues. Generally, SaaS vendors are responsible for system maintenance, back-ups, and future releases for a fixed monthly subscription fee.

SOCIAL NETWORKING

Social networking is grouping of individuals who through common Internet sites create profiles and build personal networks connecting them to other users, businesses, and organizations. Social networking is becoming a proven method for large and small practices to connect with their patients and promote the practice. The Mayo Clinic (Rochester, MN), for example, has a Facebook page that had approximately 7,000 "fans" at publication. This online presence gives them the means to communicate with patients and other fans quickly and at no cost. Their communication is then distributed among the 7,000 fans that may choose to share and distribute the clinic's message within their own personal networks, thus creating "viral" messages that have the potential to spread to millions with very little effort in a short period of time. Sites like YouTube and Twitter allow people and organizations to communicate and broadcast messages to an unlimited number of individuals and "followers."

The next generation of patients relies on and expects to communicate through social networking tools. "PatientsLikeMe" is a great example to reference (www.patientslikeme.com/). This social networking site connects patients with similar health issues or ailments.

Some businesses that have been slow to adapt to the social networking phenomenon have been penalized financially by underestimating the power of this new trend

Time Period	Method	Description
Late 1970s	Mainframe computer	Large computer that stores data while distributing and running applications (mostly designed from back office) to store and process data.
1980s	Client/server	Local servers were connected to several desktop personal computers, referred to as clients of the server.
1990s	Centralized data center or application service provider (ASP)	Basically the client/server model, with servers managed off-site.
Early 2000s	Service-oriented architecture	Similar to the off-site data center or ASP, but enables the World Wide Web to deliver software.
Mid to late 2000s	Smart client or thin client	Similar to client server model, except that it uses local central processing unit processing. The thin client emulates the server but does not have local processing. All processing is done on the server.
2010s	Software as a service (SaaS)	Technology subscriptions. Instead of servers, any computer with an Internet connection will suffice.

Table 13-2: The Evolution of Software Acquisition and Delivery

in communication. For example, when was the last time you purchased a newspaper? Some media outlets were quick to adjust their methods and include digital formats and social media tools, but most that stayed with traditional delivery methods are now suffering financially. Many print newspapers have closed their doors. Consider what the map printing business would look like today if it did not respond to the growing trend of global positioning system devices.

CONCLUSION

The key to leveraging trends is to know how and when to respond to them. You may not want to be a first adopter, but, at the same time, you also do not want to be at the end of a trend's lifecycle. Given the current state of healthcare and its dependency on health IT, trends will continue to emerge at an alarming rate. As with any new technology, refer back to Chapter 8 on procurement and negotiating to help ensure that your health IT investment is protected and the supplier is accountable for meeting your expectations.

REFERENCE

1. http://mobithinking.com/native-or-web-app. Accessed October 22, 2010.

Tools and Policies

INTRODUCTION

This appendix is devoted to a collection of resources and tools used in electronic health record (EHR) selection and implementation projects. These tools are intended to be guidelines, templates and examples of proven resources and policies—each of which can (and should) be modified to meet the needs of your practice. This chapter includes:

- Project management policies and tools
- Project staffing models
- EHR readiness assessment tools
- Vendor vetting tools
- Return-on-investment calculator
- EHR resources from the Healthcare Information and Management Systems Society

Note: The sample tools provided in this chapter are intended to assist medical practices as they undertake an EHR implementation project. Because each medical practice is different, these tools should be customized accordingly.

PROJECT MANAGEMENT POLICIES AND TOOLS

Project management is more than an efficient way of managing a new initiative. True project management requires a team effort and has its base in traditional management theory. In addition, it has become a systematic discipline that includes a unique set of tools and techniques.

This consistent set of tools, techniques and policies stems from a growing need for businesses to be able to view real-time project status and ensure that the project remains on time and within established budget parameters. The policies and tools detailed in this appendix provide concrete examples of effective processes, workflows, and procedures used by other practices during EHR adoption. This appendix is intended to serve as a reference guide for project leaders and managers.

Step One – Define Project Roles and Responsibilities

- **Physician or executive sponsor.** This individual represents the most senior level of management. He/she holds other team members accountable for project deliverables. The physician/executive sponsor signs off on project initiation and closure. This individual regularly receives project status information from project managers (e.g., progress to date, on time, on budget, critical issues). In return, he/she makes budget and resource-allocation decisions.

- **Project manager.** Usually, this individual is an experienced office leader, such as a nurse manager or team leader, who can "own" the project plan, assign resources, request and review weekly status reports (e.g., accomplishments, upcoming deliverables, issues, actual vs. baseline) and maintain project plans (e.g., create baseline, prepare reports). The project manager approves or declines updated resource requests and is responsible for reporting project status to the physician/executive sponsor and for managing the work performed by the resources. (Because the office manager/practice administrator is busy managing the practice, he/she will find it challenging to devote extra time to EHR project management. Generally, therefore, it is best to select someone other than that individual as EHR project manager.)

- **Project team members.** The project team performs work assigned to them by the project manager. Team members are responsible for reporting back to the project manager on the status of the specific tasks assigned to them, including any issues/challenges that arise. They also may be assigned the task of resolving any issues specific to their assigned tasks.

Step Two – Create Project Plan

A project plan is not complete unless it is put into writing or into a time line. This helps all project stakeholders stay on track and allows everyone to know their roles and responsibilities. A sample project plan begins on page 152.

SAMPLE PROJECT PLAN

Task/Objectives	Start Date	Finish Date	Resource by Roles and Responsibilities
Sign contract/purchase order			Customer and Vendor
Project Manager assigned (customer side/vendor side)			Customer and Vendor
Vendor to send project documentation			Vendor
Vendor to send software manuals and policies			Vendor
Project kick-off call			Customer and Vendor
Ship software and hardware			Vendor
Confirm receipt			Customer
Project Pre-Planning and Information Gathering			
Schedule kick-off meeting			Project Manager and Vendor
Review project plan and time line – make adjustments			Project Manager
Final approval of project plan and time line			Project Manager and Project Sponsor
Assigns project staff members			Project Manager and Project Sponsor
Complete implementation start-up profile			Customer
Customer information			Customer
Site location (address and name if different)			Customer
Training questionnaire			Customer
Telephone directory			Customer
Travel information			Customer
Electrical specifications (including server room)			Customer
Billable service (Outsourced?) Cable			Customer
Existing computer equipment			Customer
Lab interface specification(s) form			Customer
Specifications (patch panel)			Customer
E-mail accounts			Customer
Employee listing			Customer
Site Readiness & Installation			
Schedule pre-installation inspection			Project Manager
Install cabling if needed			Customer

Task/Objectives	Start Date	Finish Date	Resource by Roles and Responsibilities
Confirm location for workstations, servers			Customer
Install communications lines if needed			Customer
Document telephone specifications			Customer
Document electrical specifications			Customer
Document cable specifications			Customer
Document existing computer equipment			Customer
Document e-mail accounts			Customer
Identify fax server			Customer
Identify fax line			Customer
Identify/purchase modem			Customer
Identify scanner need			Customer
Identify printer need			Customer
Installation			
Test/prepare network servers			IT Support, Customer
Train customer on administrative tools			IT Support, Customer
Install SQL server or other database			IT Support, Customer
Install EHR database			IT Support, Customer
Install PM database (if applicable)			IT Support, Customer
Install customer EPM & EHRS software			IT Support, Customer
Install content tools			IT Support, Customer
Install fax manager (if applicable)			IT Support, Customer
Installation of dial-in access			IT Support, Customer
Test all of the above installed equipment			
Test and verify access to all modules			Technical Support, Project Manager, Customer
Test and verify version of EHR			Technical Support, Project Manager, Customer
Verify saved data			Technical Support, Project Manager, Customer
Verify saved images			Technical Support, Project Manager, Customer
Verify learning management tools			Technical Support, Project Manager, Customer
Verify fax manager installed			Technical Support, Project Manager, Customer

Task/Objectives	Start Date	Finish Date	Resource by Roles and Responsibilities
Verify reporting tools installed			Technical Support, Project Manager, Customer
Verify database			Technical Support, Project Manager, Customer
Verify e-mail access			Technical Support, Project Manager, Customer
Verify medication database			Technical Support, Project Manager, Customer
Confirm CPT/ICD code availability			Technical Support, Project Manager, Customer
Confirm access to customer system			Technical Support, Project Manager, Customer
Review post-installation issues			Technical Support, Project Manager, Customer
Schedule follow-up (if necessary)			Project Manager, Customer
Complete Visit Report and obtain customer signature			Technical Support, Customer
Interfaces			
Practice management and EHR interface			
Install test environment			
Schedule installation of EHR interface			Project Manager
Transfer table data from EHR			Interface Department
Inform PM interface ready for testing			Interface Department
Confirm patient demographic data in EHR			Customer, Project Manager
Confirm appointment schedules			Customer, Project Manager
Confirm charge posting to PMS			Customer, Project Manager
Interface Tested within a LIVE Environment			
Test billing interface			Interface Department
Test data from PM to EHR			Interface Department
Verify PM interface transfer complete			Interface Department
Verify patient demographic data			Customer, Project Manager
Verify appointment schedule			Customer, Project Manager

Task/Objectives	Start Date	Finish Date	Resource by Roles and Responsibilities
Verify charge posting to PM			Customer, Project Manager
Test lab interface			
Review information			Project Manager
Create documentation			Project Manager
Contact lab vendor for their specifications			Interface Manager
Assign programmer to development			Interface Manager
Determine communication link between customer and lab vendor			Interface Department, Third-party Vendor
Send documentation to programmer			Interface Manager
Test interface			Interface Manager
Test PM interface for lab charges			Interface Manager
Installation of Lab Interface LIVE Environment			
Contact lab vendor			Project Manager
Testing with lab vendor			Interface Department
Install lab vendor interface			Interface Manager, Third-party Vendor
Test PM interface for lab charges			Interface Manager, Project Manager
Train customer on use of communication link interface			Interface Manager, Project Manager
Confirm lab order processed by interface			Customer, Project Manager
Confirm lab order received properly by lab			Customer, Project Manager
Confirm lab results received properly by customer			Customer, Project Manager
Transfer of lab vendor interface			Project Manager
Transfer with lab vendor			Interface Department
Confirm communication links			Interface Department
Confirm PM transfer of LIVE environment			Interface Department
Confirm lab order processed by Interface			Customer, Project Manager
Confirm lab order received properly by lab			Customer, Project Manager
Confirm lab results received properly by EHR			Customer, Project Manager

Task/Objectives	Start Date	Finish Date	Resource by Roles and Responsibilities
Preparation for On-site			
Select training location			Customer
Scheduled training date			Customer, Project Manager
Determine attendees for training			Customer, Project Manager
Develop training content and documentation			Project Manger
EHR Training			
EHR Training			Project Manager, Implementation Specialist
System administration			Implementation Specialist, Customer
Medical records module/customer			Implementation Specialist
Patient education			Implementation Specialist, Customer
Table maintenance			Implementation Specialist, Customer
Off line document generator			Implementation Specialist, Customer
Lab assign			Implementation Specialist, Customer
Template editor			Implementation Specialist, Customer
Region editor			Implementation Specialist, Customer
Template import/export			Implementation Specialist, Customer
Document builder			Implementation Specialist, Customer
Document import/export			Implementation Specialist, Customer
Discuss database review process			Implementation Specialist
Review and verify status of staff training			Implementation Specialist, Customer
Customer and vendor confirm competition			Implementation Specialist
EHR Database Review, Modifications, Development			
Modify templates/documents			Implementation Specialist, Customer
Modify lab template			Implementation Specialist, Customer

Task/Objectives	Start Date	Finish Date	Resource by Roles and Responsibilities
Modify phone message template			Customer, Implementation Specialist
Test templates/documents			Implementation Specialist, Customer
Phase 1 templates complete			Customer, Implementation Specialist
Test system administration			Customer
Gather employee access list			Customer
Add users/assign rights based on role			Customer
Create groups/assign rights			Customer
Table Maintenance			**Customer**
Create diagnosis categories			Customer
Review/add allergies			Customer
Add employers			Customer
Add image descriptions			Customer
Add lab components			Customer
Add lab groups			Customer
Add lab tests			Customer
Add languages			Customer
Review/add medications			Customer
Create medication groups			Customer
Create modifiers categories			Customer
Assign categories to providers			Customer
Add pharmacies			Customer
Add recall type/reason			Customer
Review/add sig codes			Customer
Add/review specialty			Customer
Create service categories			Customer
Add zip code			Customer
Add zone			Customer
Prescription Report			
Forward copy of RX prescription			Customer
Forward copies of other reports			Customer
Create medication prescription report			Implementation Specialist
Install medication prescription report			Implementation Specialist
Test medication prescription report			Implementation Specialist, Customer
Review medication prescription report			Customer

Task/Objectives	Start Date	Finish Date	Resource by Roles and Responsibilities
Modify medication prescription report			Implementation Specialist
Final approval on prescription report			Customer
EHR LIVE Database			
Schedule testing			Project Manager
Copy test database to LIVE database			Customer Support
Alert project manager copy is complete			Customer Support
Confirm copy			Project Manager, Implementation Specialist, Customer
Confirm production database readiness			Project Manager, Implementation Specialist, Customer
Confirm templates available and performing correctly			Project Manager, Implementation Specialist, Customer
Confirm documents available			Project Manager, Implementation Specialist, Customer
Confirm images available and performing correctly			Project Manager, Implementation Specialist, Customer
Confirm providers available			Project Manager, Implementation Specialist, Customer
Confirm locations available			Project Manager, Implementation Specialist, Customer
Confirm appointments available			Project Manager, Implementation Specialist, Customer
Confirm e-mail functioning			Project Manager, Implementation Specialist, Customer
Confirm ability to print documents and reports			Project Manager, Implementation Specialist, Customer
Confirm ability to fax documents and reports			Project Manager, Implementation Specialist, Customer
Set location of medication prescription report			Project Manager, Implementation Specialist, Customer

Task/Objectives	Start Date	Finish Date	Resource by Roles and Responsibilities
Confirm ability to view medication report			Project Manager, Implementation Specialist, Customer
Confirm ability to print medication report			Project Manager, Implementation Specialist, Customer
Confirm ability to fax medication report			Project Manager, Implementation Specialist, Customer
Confirm ability to order labs			Project Manager, Implementation Specialist, Customer
Confirm ability to receive results			Project Manager, Implementation Specialist, Customer
EHR Training			
Key user training			Project Manager, Implementation Specialist
End user training			Project Manager, Implementation Specialist, or Customer
Go-live			Project Manager, Implementation Specialist, Customer

Step Three – Organize Implementation Processes and Tasks

Processes and tasks are organized into five major categories:

1. **Initiate.** Building a formal process to handle project-related requests is a vital step in eliminating unrealistic workloads and ad hoc resource assignments. For example, one user may request an EHR customization that could result in exceeding the project budget or allocated staff time. The ability to decide which suggestions will be implemented depends on clearly understanding the definition of a *project,* which is a *temporary* endeavor with a beginning and an end that creates a unique product or service and has interrelated activities.

2. **Analyze.** During project analysis, stakeholders and team members gather information to support formal project planning. Next, if approval to proceed is granted, they undertake budget development and other basic requirements to support project implementation. Generally, it is a good rule of thumb to adopt the vendor's budget for services and match those allocations internally with practice resources. For example, if the vendor estimates that they will need to devote 100 hours to the project, the practice should expect to do the same because someone will have to oversee vendor activities.

3. **Plan.** This project phase allows the project manager to define manageable (and measurable) pieces of work and organize them into a schedule. To plan realistically for project implementation, it is important to identify any external dependencies. For example, if a key milestone for staff training is predicated on having a training room set up, setting up these workstations may be further predicated on locating a room with enough space and power supplies. While this kind of planning may seem obvious, good project managers always account for such interdependencies and assign someone the responsibility of addressing each component sequentially. Finding out that the training room does not have adequate power supply on the day of training would be very disruptive.

4. **Execute.** This step is where "the rubber meets the road." All analyses, information gathering, and planning is now put into motion. This project phase should incorporate a well-known process called *design, build, and verify* (DBV):

    a. **Design** a rough plan for what you want the project to accomplish. This task can be done on a white board or by undertaking workflow mapping to understand how the new system is supposed to respond to end users.

    b. **Build** what you have designed.

    c. **Verify** the effectiveness of what you have designed and built, modifying it accordingly after thorough testing.

    d. Then...**implement** what you have designed, built, and tested after it is proven to work effectively.

    Using the DBV model will ensure that the project is working before the practice launches the system in a live environment. Even after implementation, DBV should be used when implementing new features, customizing existing ones or optimizing the system.

5. **Transition.** Every project must have a start and an end. A clear end to a project serves several purposes. The most important of these, however, is that a well-defined transition into go-live status gives full ownership of the system to end users. The goals of the transition should include the following:

    a. Close out the project plan.

    b. Summarize the final project status. (Although there may be a few lingering issues that require follow up, there should always be an official end to big projects like EHR system implementation. Otherwise, pending work tends to linger indefinitely.)

    c. Review the project's "lessons learned."

    d. Recognize the accomplishments of the implementation team.

    e. Celebrate!

Two critical success factors of any project are (1) to have fun and (2) be flexible. Be forewarned that many decisions in large projects have to be made with incomplete information. In addition, many good solutions are achieved only through trial and error.

Seek outside help, whenever possible, from those who have already been through this process. You may even want to consider engaging an outside expert who has experience with and knowledge of EHR implementation projects. The role of the consultant in this setting is to transfer knowledge and support practice decisions. A consultant can also act as an objective third party, which is extremely helpful during change management.

Matching t-shirts for implementation team members often help establish a "team feeling" among colleagues—in addition to generating excitement about the project for the team and the rest of staff. Make sure the implementation team has a good workroom and allow some extra time for rest. Burnout is common for people dedicated to big projects like EHR implementation, so make sure team members have some diversity in their work roles and responsibilities.

PROJECT STAFFING MODELS

Sufficient staffing levels are critical for a successful EHR implementation project. Thus, the EHR implementation team should be appropriately staffed with full-time, dedicated members who are available for team meetings, training, and conference calls. Upper-level management should immediately respond to project staffing requests, and no EHR project should move forward without proper staffing levels.

To support successful EHR implementation projects, the Healthcare Information and Management Systems Society (HIMSS) has provided estimates regarding recommended workforce levels by job description (see Table A-1).

Job Description	Staff Allocation, %
Project management	1
Management	11
Programmers	29
Operations	8
Network administration	9
Help desk	8
Personal computer support	11
Security	1
Other	22

Adapted from: IT staffing models from HIMSS Analytics April 2008 data. October 4, 2008. http://www.anticlue.net/archives/000890.htm. Accessed December 30, 2010.

Table A-1: Estimates Regarding Recommended Workforce Levels by Job Description

Staffing models can be broad, as in listing job descriptions for the project, or as detailed as naming actual people assigned to certain roles. Although the project manager's responsibility is to keep everyone on task and to ensure that work is done within certain time frames, all members of the team have equally important roles and work contiguously in their responsible roles.

It is also good to create a project staffing organization chart, as illustrated in the project staffing model below. These staffing charts may have a temporary reporting structure. For example, a technical team member may report to the CIO normally, but during the project, they would also report to the project manager. Some project members will be needed full time, while others may only participate on an as-needed basis by providing input or feedback.

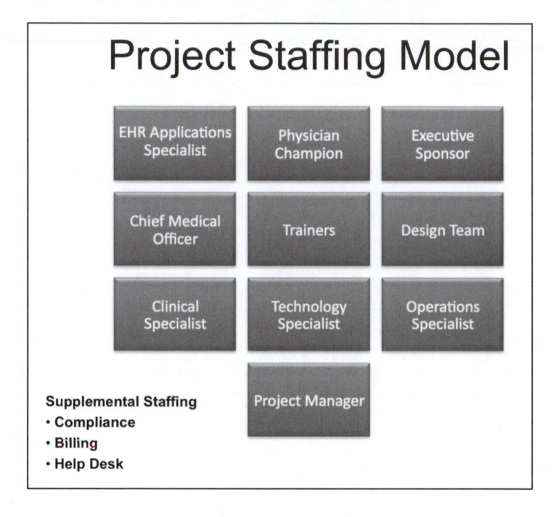

EHR READINESS-ASSESSMENT TOOLS

Readiness-assessment tools come in a variety of structures and formats. The main purpose of an EHR assessment tool is to assist in gathering the information necessary to determine how well a practice is prepared to adopt a new EHR system. The sample tool provided here includes a blend of technical and operational questions to help you establish a current baseline of practice functionality. It should also help establish the practice's EHR readiness level and clarify any outstanding requirements for technology adoption. However, because each practice is different, it is essential that you customize this guide to your practice. Thus, this tool should be used as a checklist for gathering basic information. Completing it will help you communicate more effectively with vendors, contractors, staff members and any external parties that will be assisting you with the adoption of EHR technology.

READINESS ASSESSMENT CHECKLIST

General Information

1. Practice Name: _____

2. Other Entities (Physician Network, MSO, Surgery Center, Clinic, etc.)

   _____

   _____

   _____

   _____

3. Tax Identification Number: _____

   a. If multiple TIN, Identify purpose of each:

      TIN_____

      Entity _____

      TIN_____

      Entity _____

      TIN_____

      Entity _____

4. What type of Practice? Private - Hospital-owned - Rural Health - Community-based - Urgent Care

5. Please list the specialty services provided:

   _____

   _____

   _____

   _____

6. Total Number of Physicians?_____

   Total Number of Mid-levels? _____

7. Number of locations? _____ (List Below)

Address	Number of Physicians	Number of Mid-levels

8. Other types of facilities:

   a. Diagnostic Testing Facility _____

   b. Surgery Center (ASC) _____

   c. Endoscopy Center_____

   d. Imaging Center_____

   e. Lab Service Center _____

9. Identify other services provided in the practice:

   ___ **Radiology**

   __Flat Film   __PACS   __Ultrasound   __MRI   __CT
   __Bone Density   __Other

   ___ **Laboratory (On site)**

   __Waived   __Moderate   __High Complexity
   __Phlebotomy Only

   ___ **Diagnostic Testing**

   __Endoscopy   __Pulmonary Studies   __Sleep Studies
   __Allergy Testing   __Vascular Studies   __Cardiac Studies
   __Bronchoscopy __Other _____

10. List all departments needing access to clinical documentation:

_____

_____

_____

_____

Office Accessibility

1. Do you use personal computers, "dumb" terminals or "thin" clients to access your systems with your environment? _____

2. Do all users have access to the Internet?   Yes   No

3. If you have a remote location(s)/office(s) how are the offices connected?

   Dial-up line   Leased line (56k)   T1 line   Internet connection

4. Do you currently interface with other Lab(s) or Hospital(s) systems to send and receive tests?   Yes   No

5. Lab(s) or Hospital(s) systems that you are presently interfaced with or send Lab Orders to?

   _____ Bi-directional?_____

   _____ Bi-directional?_____

   _____ Bi-directional?_____

   _____ Bi-directional?_____

6. Do you currently participate in any regional arrangement to share electronic patient level clinical data through an electronic health information exchange?

   ____ Yes, we participate and actively exchange data. The arrangement is with _____

   ____ Yes, we participate but do not exchange data. The arrangement is with _____

   ____ No, we do not have participate in any regional arrangements to share patient information.

7. Does your system use HL7 messaging for data exchange between systems?   Yes   No

8. What are your current bandwidth (please use "C") and bandwidth needs (please use "N") to support EHR?

	<5Mb/s	<15Mb/s	<25Mb/s	<50Mb/s	<75Mb/s	<75-100 Mb/s	<100Mb/s
What is your current broadband access?							
What is your minimum upstream bandwidth for a broadband connection to support HIE?							

	<5Mb/s	<15Mb/s	<25Mb/s	<50Mb/s	<75Mb/s	<75-100 Mb/s	<100Mb/s
What is your minimum downstream bandwidth for a broadband connection to support HIE?							
What is your maximum upstream bandwidth requirement for a broad-band con-nection to support HIE?							
What is your maximum downstream bandwidth requirement for a broad-band con-nection to support HIE?							

Staffing/Expense Information - Related to HIS

1. How many FTEs are dedicated to registration/check-in?_____

2. How many FTEs are dedicated to charge entry?_____

3. How many FTEs are dedicated to payment entry?_____

4. How many FTEs are dedicated to collections, self-pay and insurance?_____

5. How many FTEs are directly involved with the financial and admin-istrative aspects of the practice including staff, management, IT and clerical, but excluding physicians, clinicians, PA, NP and Residents? _____

6. To whom do you presently transmit electronic claims?
   Medicare_____   Medicaid_____
   Managed Care_____   Commercial_____

7. Are charges entered at the time of service? _____

8. If not, when are charges entered?_____

9. Does your current system provide accurate encounter tracking or missing encounter form reports?_____

10. Does your current scheduling system allow each department to set its unique scheduling parameters (i.e. type, frequency and duration)?_____

11. Do you print statements in house, or transmit them to a third party for preparation?_____

12. If you print statements in house, how often do you print?_____

13. If you transmit to a third party, how much do you pay per statement? _____

14. Do you make reminder calls for upcoming appointments?_____

15. If so, how many per month?_____

16. How many no-shows do you have on average per day?_____

17. Do you charge for no-shows?   Yes   No

18. Do you print/send recall letters or postcards?_____

19. Do you charge for medical records copying? _____
    How much?_____

20. If so, how many admissions per month?_____

21. What is the average charge for a patient visit/stay?_____

22. What is your annual revenue?_____

23. What is your total Accounts Receivable Balance?_____

24. What is your total "self-pay" A/R Balance?_____

25. What is your total "self-pay" A/R Balance over 90 days?_____

26. What is your total "Third-Party Claims" outstanding Balance?_____

27. What is your total "Third-Party Claims" outstanding balance over 90 days?_____

28. How are referral and patient letters generated? _____

29. How are test results communicated to patients?_____

30. Do you have a tracking system for identifying outstanding results and appointments?_____

31. How many FTEs are dedicated to pulling and filing patient charts? _____

32. What is the annual compensation of chart management personnel (including benefits)? _____

33. How many paper medical records do you currently maintain on site?_____

34. Do you use document storage facilities off site?_____
Annual cost of storage:_____

35. Please indicate the method for capturing clinical documentation.
Dictation / Transcription_____
Hand Write_____
Do not believe in documentation_____

36. How many FTEs are dedicated to transcription? _____

37. What is the annual compensation of transcription staff (including benefits)? _____

If you outsource transcription, what is your annual transcription cost? _____

Current EHR Information

Which of the following HIT systems are installed in your practice(s)? Include vendor name, program version and ONC Certification Level.

	Vendor	Program Version	ONC Certification
Health Information System (HIS)			
Practice Management System			
Provider Credentialing Program			
Electronic Health Record (EHR)			
Managed Care Contract Management System			
Document Imaging/Scanning			
Insurance Eligibility & Verification			
Appointment Confirmation			
Lab/Test Result Messaging			
Online Patient Registration			
Online CPT-IV, ICD-9 & HCPCS Coding Resources			
Clinical Reference Systems (CRS)			
Electronic Prescription System			
Computerized Physician Order Entry (CPOE)			

	Vendor	Program Version	ONC Certification
Lab Information System (LIS)			
Radiology Information System (RIS)			
Picture Archiving and Communication System (PACS)			

EHR Goals

1. Please list the primary reasons you want to implement an EHR System. _____

    _____

    _____

    _____

2. If you found the right system, when is your goal to be live on the EHR system? _____

3. How significant a barrier to implementation of an EHR system are the following:

	Major Barrier	Minor Barrier	Not a Barrier
Capital needed to purchase and implement			
Uncertain return on investment (ROI)			
Ongoing cost of maintaining EHR			
Resistance from physicians			
Resistance from other providers			
Resistance from staff			
Lack of capacity to select, contract and implement EHR			
Disruption in clinical care during implementation			
Lack of adequate IT staff or IT support			
Concerns about training providers and staff			
Concerns about documentation & coding			
Inappropriate disclosure of patient information			

	Major Barrier	Minor Barrier	Not a Barrier
Concerns about medical records (purging, scanning, uploading)			
Concerns about upgrades and lack of future support			

4. Which of the following models would be a preferred EHR data storage model for your practice?

   __ Federated or distributed model (all EHR data remains at practice site)

   __ Hybrid model (some copies of patient data may reside outside the practice; practice has full EHR)

   __ Centralized model (EHR data are stored centrally with a vendor/ data center)

   Need more information (please explain) _____

   _____

   _____

5. Do you have dedicated HIT professionals in your practice?
   YES   NO   (Indicate FTEs)

   _____ CIO/IT Director(s)   _____ IT Application Administrators
   _____ IT Technicians   _____ Data Warehouse Administrators/Analysts
   _____ Bio-Technicians   _____ Informatics Nurses
   _____ Other professionals trained in Informatics

6. Do you currently have a dedicated help desk system and staff for logging tickets and performing root cause analysis?
   YES   NO
   (If yes, how many FTE_____)

Hardware/Software/Projected Needs

Number of users who will use the system for access to patient information, scheduling, charge entry, payment entry, reporting and collections:

_____

Number of users who will access the EHR System for access to patient records:

Doctors _____   NP/PA _____   Nurses _____
Admin/Support Staff _____

Number of handheld devices used for clinical documentation: _____

Number of PCs installed at the nurse's stations: _____

Number of PCs installed in other clinical areas: _____

   Identify the other clinical areas: _____

Number of PCs installed at the front desk: _____

Number of PCs installed for the billing staff: _____

Number of PCs installed in other clerical areas: _____

   Identify the other clerical areas: _____

Total number of PCs in the practice (existing PCs): _____

Number of existing Windows 2000/Windows XP or higher PCs: _____

Total laser printers for printing patient information sheets, encounter forms, HCFAs, reports, etc.: _____

Total other printers for printing patient information sheets, encounter forms, HCFAs, reports, etc.: _____

Number of insurance card scanners: _____

Number of multi-purpose copiers in the practice: _____

Technical Assessment of Existing IT infrastructure:

1. Type of server presently installed (include how peripherals and terminals are connected): _____

   _____

2. What type of workstations do you have deployed? ___

   a. Type of terminals installed/number of units _____

   b. Type of PCs installed/number of units _____

   c. Type of thin clients/number of units _____

3. Version of operating system: _____

   a. On the servers? _____

   b. On the workstations? _____

4. Applications installed: _____

5. Type of hub or switch installed: _____

6. Number of ports available: _____

7. Does the site currently have access to the Internet / who is the provider / copy of statement: _____

8. Check to see if there is adequate power supply at the Dmarc location and at PC location _____

9. Printers and type: _____

   Type of cabling installed: _____

10. Who is currently supporting your infrastructure? _____

11. How do you back-up your current system? _____

12. Describe your disaster recovery/business continuity plan. _____

_____

_____

_____

_____

VENDOR VETTING TOOLS

This section provides several sample tools to assist medical practices with vendor selection. These tools include samples of the following documents:

- Request for information
- Request for proposal
- Vendor profile
- Vendor demonstration script
- Vendor demonstration scorecard
- Practice site visit checklist
- List of questions for vendor reference checks

Request for Information

Before diving deeply into vendor vetting, it is sometimes helpful to begin with gathering basic information about potential vendors. A request for information (RFI) is usually a one- or two-page letter sent to multiple vendors requesting information about their products and services (see page 176). The results of the RFI are used to weed out vendors that may not meet a practice's basic EHR requirements. You may want to state the practice's minimum requirements so you do not waste your time or that of the vendors. For example, adding a statement that indicates *vendors must be CCHIT certified* will eliminate any EHR solution that is not eligible for federal funding through the American Recovery and Reinvestment Act of 2009 or other government initiatives.

Request for Proposal

A request for proposal (RFP) is a document that comprehensively describes a client's functional requirements to potential vendors (see pages 177–182). Each potential vendor completes the same document, allowing the client an opportunity to compare/contrast vendors based on their ability to meet the client's clear and specific requirements.

An RFP should be written clearly and concisely so that vendor response teams do not have to guess about any of the client's requirements. It is recommended that RFP writers use simple terms (e.g., "use" instead of "utilize") and direct questions. The goal when writing an RFP is to be clear so that the responses one receives are as precise as possible.

Vendor Profile

One of the essential strategies for selection of an EHR is to research potential vendors. Even prior to setting up a vendor demonstration, you will want to find out how long they have been in business, get an overview of their financial stability, and assess their commitment to research and development. The Vendor Profile – A to Z is a helpful tool for learning what you need to know about potential vendors (see pages 183–184).

SAMPLE REQUEST FOR INFORMATION (RFI)

Dear Vendor _____

This Request for Information (RFI) is for information only. It does not con-
stitute a solicitation for bids or an offer of a contract. Responses will not
bind the vendor contractually or monetarily, or in any other way, but will
provide _____ with information and comparables if the Practice does go forward with a Request for Proposal (RFP). It is the intention
of the Practice to generate an RFP based on information received from
this RFI.

Responders are requested to:

1. Supply a brief corporate overview.
2. Send marketing brochures, demo disk and other information to
    education us on your products and services.
3. No unsolicited information over the telephone at this time.
4. Number of systems installed in the state of _____.
5. Number of systems installed in practices over _____ providers.
6. Number of systems installed in _____ (state specialty).

Please submit your responses to _____ at the address
below.

Responses must be received by _____

Questions and comments should be directed to _____

SAMPLE REQUEST FOR PROPOSAL (RFP)

ABC Medical Practice
Anywhere USA

ELECTRONIC HEALTH RECORDS
REQUEST FOR PROPOSAL

I. INTRODUCTION AND OVERVIEW OF ABC Medical Practice

ABC Medical Practice is soliciting proposals from vendors of electronic health records.

ABC Medical Practice consists of 5 physicians and 2 mid-levels providing expertise in diagnosis, evaluation and management of digestive disease for patients in _____. The practice owns and operates a surgery center and has two satellite offices. We have 30 concurrent system users. The target effective date for implementation of the electronic health record system is _____.

ABC Medical Practice has identified the following functional requirements for the electronic medical records systems:
- Integrated billing _____ Practice Management system
- Template development with the ability to be customized
- Reporting tools
- E & M coding and auditing
- Prescription refill processing (including allergy reference and interactions)
- Integration with Microsoft

II. INSTRUCTIONS TO RESPONDER

A. SELECTION APPROACH

Responses to this RFP will be evaluated and used as the basis for selecting vendors to proceed through the remainder of the selection process, including detailed product functionality review and demonstrations, reference checks and site visits.

Vendor responses to this RFP will be evaluated against criteria that include:
- *Quality of response* - for completeness and overall quality of the vendor's response, including submission of appropriate and reasonable responses to all questions throughout this RFP.
- *Vendor stability* - the demonstrated financial stability and viability of the vendor's organization.

- **Vendor experience** - the proven ability of the vendor organization to deliver, implement and support the proposed product and similar healthcare and information system environments.
- **Application functionality** - the proposed product's sophistication and functionality.
- **Interface capabilities** - the ability to interface effectively with existing and planned information systems environment and with third-party systems.
- **System cost** - the overall one-time and ongoing costs associated with the proposed applications, hardware, implementation, customization, interfacing, conversion and support services.

B. <u>SELECTION SCHEDULE</u>

The anticipated time line for this system selection process is as follows:

ACTIVITY	DATE
Issue RFP	June 1
Vendor RFP Responses Due	June 15
Site Visits	June 22-26
Select Electronic Health Record System	June 30

C. <u>RFP RESPONSES DESTINATION</u>

One original and six copies of the response must be received no later than 5:00 PM, Pacific Daylight Time (PDT), on _____, and must be delivered to:

> Mrs. Office Manager
> 1234 Medical Office Lane
> Anywhere, USA 11111
>
> (999) 999-9999
> officemanager@ABCmedical.com

All questions pertaining to the RFP and product evaluation process should be forwarded to Mrs. Office Manager at the address listed above.

D. INSTRUCTIONS FOR VENDOR RESPONSE

Responses must meet the following format requirements:
- Responses should not exceed 20 pages (excluding cover letter and attachments).
- Response to each question should follow the same outline as the requested information.
- Additional requested information should be clearly labeled and submitted as attachments to the response.

- Any promotional materials and other documents not specifically requested by this RFP may also be submitted as attachments to the response.

III. VENDOR RESPONSE

A. CORPORATE INFORMATION

1. Identifying information:
   - Provide the name, address and telephone number of the legal entity(ies) with which any contract would be written.
   - Specify your incorporation structure.
   - Years in business.

2. Provide the location of the office that would provide implementation and support services to ABC Medical Practice.

3. Provide the location of the office that conducts product development.

B. FINANCIAL INFORMATION

Submit a copy of your most recent audited financial statement, or similar information that clearly substantiates the current and ongoing financial condition of the company, including the following comparative information for your company for each of the past three years:
- Total sales
- Net income
- Assets and liabilities
- Number of employees

C. STAFF RESUMES

Provide resumés, not exceeding two pages each, of the staff to be assigned to this contract. Resumés should contain the following information and qualifications of staff who would work on the project:
- Name
- Position description, title and areas of responsibility with respect to the quoted work
- Relationship and tenure to your firm: full-time/part-time, officer or employee, subcontractor or other relationship
- Summary of qualifications of the individual staff, including particular skills, length of experience, significant accomplishments and other pertinent information

D. CLIENT BASE AND REFERENCES

1. Provide a minimum of five references, with size and demographic profiles similar to those of ABC Medical Practice, currently using the product and release you are proposing. Reference information should include:
   - Organization name, location, and type
   - Name, title and telephone and fax number of an authorized contact
   - Description of practice management system interfaces
   - The date production usage of the system began
   - Operational statistics, such as number of lives, providers, specialties, etc.
   - Release or version number of software implemented

2. How many organizations are currently using the proposed application (and specific release) in a production environment?
   - Number of systems sold
   - Number of current users

E. CONTRACT TERMINATION FOR DEFAULT

Indicate if your company has had a contract terminated for default in the last five years. Termination for default is defined as *notice to stop performance due to your firm's nonperformance or poor performance*. If your firm has had a contract terminated for default in this period, then submit full details, including the other party's name, address and phone number.

F. APPLICATION DESCRIPTION AND FUNCTIONALITY

1. Specify the name, the release number and release date of the application you are proposing for ABC Medical Practice.

2. Describe the modules available and the primary functionality of each component or module.

3. Specify any product component or modules that are not fully integrated with the core applications and explain how information is shared.

4. Describe the reporting functionality available with the applications. Describe the options for selecting the data elements and specific selection and sorting criteria.

5. Describe the key features of your product that differentiates it from competitive products.

6. Attach copies of main menu and data entry screens.

7. Maximum number of users that can log on to the system at once.

8. Product focus (size of group).

G. DATA CONVERSION

ABC Medical Practice would like to convert its data from its transcription company. Describe your approach to converting data into your system.

H. <u>UPGRADES AND NEW RELEASES</u>

Describe your approach to upgrades, new releases and system enhancements. Are upgrades included as part of the purchase price or maintenance fee? How frequently do you issue upgrades and new releases? How does your system update CPT codes, RVU and ICD information? What is the cost (if any) to users for system upgrades?

I. <u>TECHNICAL ARCHITECTURE</u>

1. Describe the technical architecture of the applications/modules you would propose for ABC Medical Practice. Include details on the data architecture, programming language, available hardware/network environments, and minimum workstation requirements.

2. Specify the technical configuration you would recommend for ABC Medical Practice. Include server, workstation, network, communications and user interface components. Recommend how it will be installed on our current server.

3. Describe the amount of downtime experienced by users in the last 12 months.

4. Describe the import and export utilities available with your applications that support interfacing with physician practice, hospital, and health plan systems. Specify the EDI standards to which your software adheres.

5. Describe the methods (i.e., tools) available to generate both standard and ad hoc reports. Specify compatibility with voice recognition software.

J. <u>IMPLEMENTATION AND SUPPORT SERVICES</u>

1. Attach a sample implementation work plan for the products that you are proposing to ABC Medical Practice.

2. Describe your approach to on-site training.

3. Provide a sample of the training manual that covers creating reports.

4. Include a sample of the user documentation that supports the same function specified in the prior question.

5. Specify the office location of resources that would be providing implementation services, training, and ongoing application support. What are the hours of operation?

6. Estimation of the time to proficiency for users.

K. COST INFORMATION

1. Provide a detailed cost estimate for the full implementation of the products you are proposing to ABC Medical Practice. Include line items for license fees for application modules and recommended tools, interfaces, computer hardware and peripherals (servers, workstations, printers etc.), networking/communications, implementation services, training services, and ongoing support. Clearly highlight the areas for which you provide support, the basis of the support, and the annual costs based on the proposed solution for ABC Medical Practice. What additional products (if any) are not included in the prices above, but are available at an extra charge to enhance the basic system?

2. Of the above components for which you provided cost information, specify the components (i.e., PCs) and/or support that ABC Medical Practice may acquire from other sources.

L. ONC Certification Compliance

1. Does your EHR meet ONC Certification compliance requirements necessary to qualify for EHR incentive payments?

2. If Yes, which version?

3. Will you provide a written guarantee to conform to all current and future ONC certification compliance requirements?

VENDOR PROFILE
A TO Z

A. Company name	
B. Address (city, state zip code)	
C. Contact name	
D. Contact phone number	
E. Contact fax number	
F. Contact E-mail address	
G. Company website	
H. Annual company revenue	
I. Years in business	
J. Years selling EHR systems	
K. Total number of physicians (not users) using EHR	
L. Total number of [Specialty] using EHR	
M. List all products/solutions.	
N. Provide three references.	(1)
	(2)
	(3)
O. Payment and licensing terms	
• Are maintenance fees included?	
• How do you charge for maintenance (e.g., percentage of total software cost, fixed fee, usage)?	
• How are licenses issued (e.g., per user/provider/sign-on, etc.)?	
• Please specify license/agreement type (e.g., purchase agreement, term license, software as services).	
• What are the standard payment terms?	

• Can payment terms be based on project milestones or accomplishments?	
• Is training included in the EHR's base cost? What type of training is available (e.g., Web-based, on-site, classroom)?	
P. Are there discounts for staff members who become certified in software use?	
Q. List any user groups.	
R. Describe your system warranty.	
S. Do you provide any performance guarantees?	
T. How are defects, bugs, and client disputes resolved?	
U. Frequency of upgrades	
V. Does your company provide unlimited upgrades and future enhancements?	
W. Is your EHR system certified to meet current compliance standards?	
X. Does your company provide a stimulus-compliance guarantee?	
Y. Does your system conform to our state/commonwealth HIE?	
Z. What are the terms for termination? In the event of contract termination, how is data converted?	

Vendor Demonstration Script

Every vendor comes well prepared to demonstrate how they believe their product works in a clinical setting. Vendors use a demonstration script that they have written in advance. Vendor-prepared demonstration scripts are designed to work flawlessly and highlight the program's best features. While their planned (and well-rehearsed) demonstration is interesting and useful, it is generally wise to ask a vendor to use a demonstration script that has been developed specifically to demonstrate how their product will work in your practice.

A customized vendor demonstration script is perhaps one of the best tools to help you evaluate the solutions offered by each vendor in an apples-to-apples comparison. In addition, it will demonstrate the vendor's ability to be flexible "on the fly."

For example, the first vendor you see may struggle to get through your practice's customized demonstration script because his/her system is incomplete, whereas a more qualified vendor breezes through it because his/her system is more comprehensive. Without a customized demonstration script, you will see only what the vendor wants you to see—and it is guaranteed that their script will make their system look very good.

Vendor Demo Script				
VENDOR DEMO **General Visit, health maintenance alerts, lab request, e-script, Coding**				
Patient name	Earnie Baker		ESTABLISHED PATIENT	
Date of Service	today			
Demographics	Male, non-smoker			
	(address, etc. - whatever you want)			
Medical history	Medical History: arthritis, hypertension. Medication List: Zocor 40mg QD, Hydrochlorothiazide 50mg QD, Celebrex 200mg QD, Allergic to penicillin: Prior BP 130/80, Pulse 85, Weight 160, Height 69"			
CHIEF COMPLAINT	Frequent urination and burning			
Venue / Stage of Process	**User**		**Interaction with system**	**Comments**
Ambulatory Clinic				
Patient Care	RN or MA	1	RN/MA asks initial assessment questions. Pt states that he has noticed frequent urination for past 3 weeks. In past 5 days, there is some burning. (office lab processing UA & sending specimen for culture) No blood. Vital signs, Wt 167, BP 152/94, Pulse 80.	
	RN or MA		During review, nurse sees health maintenance alert that patient is past due for PSA. She advises patient.	
Patient Care	Doctor-Exam	2	On examination - Well developed, well nourished, slight tenderness in abdomen, no edema of legs or feet.	Demo system's charting methodology, mention lab interfaces
	Doctor-Assessment/Plan	3	1. Probable UTI, write script for ampicillin; changed script to Cipro 2. Order urine culture	System presents drug allergy alert
		4	Diagnosis: Urinary Tract Infection, suspected	
E&M	Doctor-reviews coding	5	Review E&M coding, automatic coding, etc., how EMR can help prevent missed charges, etc.	

Vendor Demonstration Scorecard

An essential tool for vetting vendors is a demonstration scorecard (see pages 187–188). Vendor demonstrations may be scheduled to take place during several weeks, each presentation lasting three to four hours. The scorecard helps you keep track of your likes and dislikes as each vendor presents their EHR product. Without a scorecard, it can be easy to forget or confuse important features about each product/vendor. The scorecard is also a great way to help your selection committee build a consensus toward a preferred vendor based on defined objectives and overall performance. Without this tool, members of the selection committee can be delayed by debating options and sometimes make poor decisions, especially when there is someone who can easily influence opinion without justification.

Practice Site Visit Tool

When conducting practice site visits, we recommend the use of a checklist (see pages 189–190). This tool will help you remain consistent when capturing information, allowing you to make an apples-to-apples comparison of products/services later.

Vendor Reference Questions

One of the final and most important steps in making a good vendor decision is to conduct reference checks. Here is a list of questions to consider asking when contacting vendor references:

- What were the top five reasons your practice selected the software?
- How did the software perform vs. expectations?
- What was the quality of staff training provided by the vendor?
- What was the quality of the vendor's implementation team?
- Did the vendor meet deadlines?
- Did the vendor stay on budget?
- What was the general attitude of vendor staff (e.g., friendly, adversarial)?
- How did the vendor deal with any problems that arose during implementation?
- Did your practice receive a satisfactory resolution to those problems?
- Have there been any system defects? If so, how were they corrected?
- Does the vendor respond to staff issues/concerns in a timely manner?
- What are the top five major benefits of the software?
- What are the top five major limitations of the software?
- Were there any hidden or unexpected costs?
- How were interfaces handled?
- Did you do a data conversion? Was it successful?
- How did the vendor respond to any difficulties?
- What other vendors did you consider? Why did you not select them?
- If you had to do it over again, would you still choose the same vendor?

VENDOR DEMONSTRATION SCORE CARD

Rating Scale

1: Poor	2: Below Average	3: Adequate	4: Good	5: Excellent

Please rate the vendor presentations based on the above rating scale.

Characteristics and Qualities	Vendor 1	Vendor 2
Your impression based on their corporate overview		
Your impression based on their accomplishments		
Your impression of the appearance of the application (design, workflow)		
Will support/improve your job		
Ease of use (easy to understand the workflow)		
Ability to improve reimbursement		
Layout of the screen, navigation accessibility of information		
Ease of interoffice communication (i.e., Physician-Nurse/Nurse-Receptionist...)		
Ease of data entry		
Overall workflow efficiency		
Ability to deliver/improve the quality of care		
Overall impression of the application		
TOTAL		

Comments

Vendor 1 positives

_____

_____

Vendor 1 negatives

_____

_____

Vendor 2 positives

_____

_____

Vendor 2 negatives

_____

_____

SAMPLE SITE VISIT TOOL

Who is Representing: ❑ Information Technology ❑ Physicians ❑ Ancillaries ❑ Patient Care/Management ❑ Registration ❑ Health Information ❑ Pharmacy ❑ Other: _____

Who did you meet with:

Contact name: _____   Phone: _____

Email: _____   Dept: _____

Key Observations

1. Functionality review by department:

2. User training: How much? Was it enough?

3. Implementation time line (what came up and when)?

4. How much was customized by the vendor or the customer? Who did the customization?

5. Did they get what they thought they would get?

Overall Observations

6. How similar was the software to what was demonstrated?

7. How broadly was the system being used?

8. What were the lessons learned?

9. What were the surprises?

10. What were the goals of the facility and were these achieved?

11. How much scheduled/unscheduled downtime?

12. How does this system help communication between departments?

13. How does this system assist with following policies and procedures?

Department Functionality

14. What specific department functionality is being used?

15. What is still done manually and why?

16. What reports are you receiving?

17. What works well and what works poorly?

18. What are you planning to change?

19. Was the vendor's staff helpful for the department during implementation?

20. How flexible are screens, forms and reports?

21. How responsive is the system (speed)?

22. How much help is available online?

23. After a downtime, what information must be re-entered into the system?

24. Has the system made your job easier?

RETURN-ON-INVESTMENT CALCULATOR

Return on investment (ROI) analysis is a tool that is commonly used to measure the financial benefits/gains of adopting a new project.

When completing an ROI analysis before EHR implementation, you will be required to make certain assumptions to use this tool. We recommend using conservative assumptions to avoid misrepresenting the project's financial benefits. Conservative assumptions will also ensure that you have properly evaluated the project's hard and soft costs. For example, although it is easy to estimate the cost of the software because the vendor will provide you with a written price quote, estimating the cost of lost physician productivity is a bit more challenging. Some productivity loss will inevitably occur; thus, it is best to predict the worst-case scenario to avoid setting unrealistic expectations. For example, because it is common to see a 20 to 30 percent reduction in physician productivity during the first four to six weeks of EHR implementation, it is wise for the practice to budget accordingly. Also, it is important to capture miscellaneous expenses, such as cabling, travel expenses and extra equipment. You may also want to add approximately 10 percent of the project's total cost to assist in addressing any unexpected circumstances.

PRACTICE NAME: xxxx	YEAR	YEAR		
	Before EMR Implementation	**After EMR Implementation**	**Difference**	**Percent Difference**
Number of FTE - Providers	5	5	0	0.00%
Number of FTE Mid-levels	1	1	0	0.00%
Total Providers	6	6	0	0.00%
Number of Admin Staff	12	10	(2)	-16.67%
Number of Clinical Staff	6	6	0	0.00%
Total Annual Charges	$ 6,000,000.00	$ 7,440,000.00	$ 1,440,000.00	24.00%
Total Charges per Month	$ 500,000.00	$ 620,000.00	$ 120,000.00	24.00%
Charges per Provider per Month	$ 83,333.33	$ 103,333.33	$ 20,000.00	24.00%
Charges per Provider per Day (21 business days per month)	$ 3,968.25	$ 4,920.63	$ 952.38	24.00%
Total Patient Visits per month (Doctors)	2500	2550	50	2.00%
Patient Visits per Provider per Month	417	425	8	2.00%
Patient Visits per Provider per Day (21 business days per month)	20	20	0	2.00%
Current Insurance Aging	$ 400,000.00	$ 380,000.00	$ (20,000.00)	-5.00%
30 to 60 Insurance Aging	$ 150,000.00	$ 140,000.00	$ (10,000.00)	-6.67%
60 to 90 Insurance Aging	$ 185,000.00	$ 80,000.00	$ (105,000.00)	-56.76%
90 to 120 Insurance Aging	$ 35,000.00	$ 50,000.00	$ (5,000.00)	-9.09%
120 plus Insurance Aging	$ 20,000.00			
TOTAL INSURANCE AGING	$ 790,000.00	$ 650,000.00	$ (140,000.00)	-17.72%
Current Patient Aging	$ 40,000.00	$ 38,000.00	$ (2,000.00)	-5.00%
30 to 60 Patient Aging	$ 25,000.00	$ 23,000.00	$ (2,000.00)	-8.00%
60 to 90 Patient Aging	$ 15,000.00	$ 10,000.00	$ (5,000.00)	-33.33%
90 to 120 Patient Aging	$ 12,000.00	$ 26,000.00	$ (1,000.00)	-3.70%
120 plus Patient Aging	$ 15,000.00			
TOTAL PATIENT AGING	$ 107,000.00	$ 97,000.00	$ (10,000.00)	-9.35%
TOTAL ACCOUNTS RECEIVABLE	$ 897,000.00	$ 747,000.00	$ (150,000.00)	-16.72%
Accounts Receivable per Provider	$ 149,500.00	$ 124,500.00	$ (25,000.00)	-16.72%
How many new patients do you see daily?	16			
Business days per year (12*21)	252			
TOTAL NEW PATIENTS	4032			
Chart Cost ($3 per new paper chart)	$ 12,096.00	savings		
Cost Savings for not purchasing additional chart rack after EMR implementation	x	savings		
What was/is your annual transcription costs?	$ 61,000.00	$ 5,000.00	$ (56,000.00)	-91.80%
Transcription Cost per Provider (Annual)	$ 10,166.67	$ 833.33	$ (9,333.33)	-91.80%
Transcription Cost per Provider (Monthly)	$ 847.22	$ 69.44	$ (777.78)	-91.80%

EHR RESOURCES FROM HIMSS

Several available EHR implementation tools are designed for a dynamic environment so they can address evolving policies and regulations as well as frequent shifts in the health IT landscape. As a result, HIMSS has provided various dynamic EHR evaluation tools on its website.

HIMSS Ambulatory Information Systems

Health IT adoption is indispensable in efforts to improve the quality of patient care. HIMSS is at the forefront of health IT adoption, and its Ambulatory Information Steering Committee (AISC) fosters an active community that constantly develops new tools. To learn more about health IT adoption, see www.himss.org/ASP/topics_ ambulatorycare.asp. To join AISC and related groups, please contact Mary Griskewicz, Senior Director, Ambulatory Information Systems, HIMSS, at mgriskewicz@himss.org.

Conducting an Effective EHR Demonstration for the Ambulatory Practice

www.himss.org/content/files/ConductingEffectiveEHRDemonstration.pdf
This tool assists HIMSS members in evaluating EHR software systems/modules in preparation for stage one Meaningful Use. HIMSS encourages members to use this rating scale as a starting point for making informed EHR decisions.

The Digital Office

www.himss.org/ASP/topics_FocusDynamic.asp?faid=155
The Digital Office, a complimentary monthly eNewsletter, connects medical practices, clinics and community health centers with the latest information on health IT and EHRs. Published the last Wednesday of each month, *The Digital Office* is a valuable resource for all HIMSS members, physicians, the media and anyone involved and interested in the transformation of today's medical practice through health IT.

EHR Brochures for Medical Professionals

HIMSS regularly produces informational brochures on topics of interest to members. Among these are:
- Getting Started with an EMR
  www.himss.org/content/files/GettingStartedEMR_Flyer1.pdf
- Selecting the Right EMR Vendor
  www.himss.org/content/files/SelectingEMR_Flyer2.pdf
- The Legal Electronic Medical Record
  www.himss.org/content/files/LegalEMR_Flyer3.pdf
- Connecting a Diagnostic Medical Device with Your EMR
  www.himss.org/content/files/ConnectMedDeviceEMRFlyer4.pdf

EHR Implementation Success Factors for Your Medical Practice

www.himss.org/content/files/20101007-1-5-doc-implementation-success-factors-FINAL.pdf
www.himss.org/content/files/201010076-6-10-doc-implementation-success-factors-FINAL.pdf
These documents offer guidelines on how to execute a smart implementation process. Whether an ambulatory practice has up to five physicians or between six and ten physicians, these documents provider specific recommendations to help practices through the EMR implementation process.

Electronic Health Record Incentive Program (Temporary Certification): What Eligible Professionals Need to Know fact sheet

www.himss.org/content/files/TemporaryCertification.pdf
Published in September 2010, this series of informational papers explores various topics surrounding Meaningful Use, Certification Criteria, Standards and Implementation Specifications. The information in these papers is offered as a starting point for making informed decisions about implementing a certified EHR.

EHR Readiness Toolkit

www.himss.org/ASP/topics_FocusDynamic.asp?faid=421
This HIMSS toolkit provides ambulatory practice owners, administrators and IT staff with practical tools and resources to assess practice needs, including the steps required to determine practice readiness for successful EHR implementation.

EMR Return-on-Investment Calculator

www.himss.org/ASP/ROI_Calc.asp
This calculator provides a high level view of potential benefits and costs associated with implementing an ambulatory EMR solution for a private physician practice or at a community health center. The calculator is designed as an "easy to use and understand" first step toward a more formal cost/benefit analysis.

HIMSS E-Prescribing

https://himsseprescribingwiki.pbworks.com/w/page/18288936/FrontPage?faid=335&tid=11
This wiki helps promote collaboration among organizations that are implementing electronic prescribing (E-prescribing) interfaces. HIMSS encourages members to share their experiences and collaborate with colleagues.

HIMSS eLearning Academy

www.himss.org/asp/educationHome.asp
HIMSS eLearning Academy is a Web-based, online learning system offering a wide range of educational sessions and courses, including many focused on EHR implementation. Education offerings include education sessions presented at HIMSS' Annual Conference and Exhibition and Virtual Conference and Expo.

Meaningful Use OneSource

www.himss.org/ASP/topics_meaningfuluse.asp

Meaningful Use OneSource is a repository of hundreds of documents, tools and links to other knowledge available on the Internet. This authoritative knowledge resource equips users to prepare for the Meaningful Use and Certification Criteria and Standards regulations; it offers answers on how to meet the meaningful use and certification criteria and how to receive the Medicare and Medicaid incentive funding. Resources include recently released updates on federal and state laws and regulations, updated Web links and new podcasts.

Nicholas E. Davies Awards of Excellence

www.himss.org/davies/index.asp

The Nicholas E. Davies Awards of Excellence, sponsored by HIMSS, recognize excellence in the implementation and value derived from EHRs. The HIMSS Davies Awards honor healthcare organizations in four categories: organizational, ambulatory care, community health organizations and public health. The Davies Award website features business cases on EHR best practices, ROI, and "lessons learned" for ambulatory care practices, community health centers, hospitals and public health institutions.

Quality 101

www.himss.org/ASP/topics_patientSafety.asp

This online portal of tools and resources, developed by the HIMSS Patient Safety & Quality Outcomes Committee, provides an introduction to the growing field of quality measures, standards of care, and evidence-based medicine.

Defining and Testing EMR Usability:
Principles and Proposed Methods of EMR Usability Evaluation and Rating

www.himss.org/content/files/HIMSS_DefiningandTestingEMRUsability.pdf

Developed in June 2009 by the HIMSS EHR Usability Task Force, this document explores usability principles applicable to EMRs. The authors describe methods of usability evaluation, offering ways to measure efficiency and effectiveness, including patient safety. Samples of objective, cost-efficient test scenarios for evaluating EMR usability as an adjunct to certification are included.

Acronyms Used in This Book

AAFP	American Association of Family Physicians
ACO	accountable care organization
ACR-NEMA	American College of Radiology - National Electrical Manufacturers Association
ACSII	American Standard Code for Information Interchange
AHIMA	American Health Information Management Association
Alliance	National Alliance for Health Information Technology
AMA	American Medical Association
AMIA	American Medical Informatics Association
ANSI	American National Standards Institute
ARRA	American Recovery and Reinvestment Act of 2009
ASC	Accredited Standards Committee
ASO	Accredited Standards Organization
ASP	application service provider
ASTM	American Society for Testing and Materials
ATA	American Telemedicine Association
CAH	critical access hospital
CCHIT	Certification Commission for Health Information Technology
CCHITT	International Telegraph & Telephone Consultative Committee
CCOW	Clinical Context Object Workgroup
CDC	Centers for Disease Control and Prevention
CEN	Committee European De Normalization
CEO	chief executive officer
CHIP	Children's Health Insurance Program
CMO	chief medical officer
CMS	Centers for Medicare & Medicaid Services

CNM	certified nurse-midwife
CPOE	computerized practitioner order entry
CPRI	Computer-based Patient Record Institute
DBV	design, build, and validation
DIMS	document imaging management system
EDI	electronic data interchange
EHR	electronic health record
E-prescribing	electronic prescribing
EP	eligible professional
ERD	entity relationship diagram
FQHC	Federally Qualified Health Center
HIE	health information exchange
HIMA	Health Industry Manufacturers Association
HIMSS	Healthcare Information and Management Systems Society
HIPAA	Health Insurance Portability and Accountability Act of 1996
HIS	hospital information system
HISB	ANSI Healthcare Information Standards Board
HITECH	Health Information Technology for Economic and Clinical Health Act of 2009
HIT PAPD	A Health Information Technology Planning Advance Planning Document
IEEE	Institute of Electrical & Electronic Engineers
IHI	Institute for Health Improvement
IP	Internet protocol address
ISO	International Organization for Standardization
IT	information technology
JHITA	Joint Healthcare Information Technology Alliance
MAO	Medicare Advantage Organization
MGMA	Medical Group Management Association
MRI	Medical Records Institute
NCPDP	National Council for Prescription Drug Programs
NPI	National Provider Identifier
NPPES	National Plan and Provider Enumeration System
ONC	Office of the National Coordinator for Health Information Technology
ONC-ATCB	ONC-Authorized Testing and Certification Body
PA	physician assistant

PACS	picture archiving and communication system
PC	personal computer
PDA	personal digital assistant
PECOS	Provider Enrollment, Chain and Ownership System
PHR	personal health record
PM	practice management
PQRI	Physicians Quality Reporting Initiative
RFI	request for information
RFP	request for proposal
RHC	rural health clinic
RHIO	regional health information organization
ROI	return on investment
RTF	rich text format
SaaS	software as a service
SNOMED CT	Systematized Nomenclature of Medicine - Clinical Terms
SME	subject matter expert
VPN	virtual private network
WEDI	Workgroup for Electronic Data Interchange

Index